Three Voices

By

Lesley Hawkins

To Mum

I will not say goodbye cause you're not gone,
I shall feel you every morning
When I turn and stretch to face the sun.
When I stride across the fields with chasing dogs
And the wind whips through my hair,
I'll know you feel it too
As you are there.

I'll greet the crows and pigeons when they land
And pause to hear their messages,
Sometimes I will listen, sometimes not
As that is how it always is with us.
I'll find you in the tangle of my garden
And smell you in its fragrant, heady blooms.
You'll be there when I choose
Between the gooey, sweet meringue and the healthy, crunchy
apple,
Telling me, 'Moderation in all things'
And I'll choose both.

I'll greet each new adventure with a smile
However much I quake on the inside,
As you did and fooled us all.
When I'm burdened with too much to do
Yet my children need my ears,
I'll know most things can wait
But love can't
As you showed me.

When they graduate, marry or perform
You'll sit beside me beaming your bright smile.
Yet when they fall, as fall they must
I'll pick them up, console and set them on their way
As you did me.
I'll see you in the eyes of my children's children
And I promise I will love them as fiercely and as gently
As you have mine.

For as long as there is them and me and us
You are not gone
You'll always be my mum
And I promise you
I'll dance.

Foreword

I wrote this book to help me cope while I managed my mother's care, as she struggled with dementia. Like Katie I have three children and work as a teacher. That is where the similarities end. This is not our story; this is a work of fiction. However, the themes are all too real. Dementia is our nation's biggest killer, its far-ranging impact damaging relationships and destroying families. The voices of those afflicted by it are seldom heard, as they are too busy trying to survive. This book is my attempt to speak out on their behalf.

Chapter 1

Beginnings

The door was shut. The dog was inside so that was OK. Where was her coat? She needed her coat. She had better go inside and get it. The door was shut. The dog was safe inside so that was OK.

She looked at her feet. She was wearing her slippers. Why? She needed her shoes. She had better put them on. The door was shut. Why? The dog was safe inside, so it was OK. She was cold. She needed her coat. She had better put it on. The door was shut. The dog was safe, so it was OK.

She shivered.

At work Katie felt her phone buzz in her pocket. Her first thought was thank goodness she had switched it to vibrate. What if it was important? She glanced at the classroom assistant. She knew she couldn't trust her yet. Not two weeks into the job. Checking a phone during class time was an absolute no. She steeled herself to ignore the persistent ringing and looked back at the child sitting next to her.

"Come on Bluebell-Rose let's break it down, b-e-d what does that make." Bluebell -Rose looked at her blankly. The phone buzzed again.

"B-e-d, try and blend the sounds together."

"Bed!" said Bluebell-Rose triumphantly.

"That's right! Now try the sentence again."

Bluebell-Rose's face contorted as she starred at "go" the word she had managed to read just one minute ago.

Joan was cold. The door was still shut. The dog was still safe, yet somehow her shoes and coat were the other side of the door. She couldn't open it. The other thing she needed was also the other side. She couldn't remember what that was, although she knew it was important. Katie's face swam into her head. That's it! Katie would know the answer. How was she to find Katie? She started to walk.

Break time had arrived at last and Katie had checked her phone. It was only Jack's number. That could wait. He was always forgetting she was back at work and ringing to complain about something. She slipped her phone into her handbag and locked it away in her desk. No more distractions! She needed to nail this job. She sat in the staffroom slipping her coffee.

"So how are you finding foundation class?" It was the deputy head; best be on her guard. However, she couldn't pretend all was well, as she would see through that in a second.

"To be honest while it is very different to year 3, I feel I am getting there. I got Bluebell-Rose to read a whole sentence to me today. She shows signs of learning difficulties, although I think it is probably lack of exposure to books at home. She shows poor social skills too." That was an understatement. The child could barely string a sentence together, had no idea how to use a knife and fork or how to play with other children. She only became animated when the tablets came out. Those she could use with remarkable dexterity.

The deputy head was smiling. "I think you are right. And I think you will settle in well here. Don't be afraid to ask for help. We have all had to restart our careers at some point and know how hard it is to adapt at first."

Katie smiled back knowing that the praise wasn't just based on her assessment of one problem child. Her extra hours of preparation had been noted. And at the end of the day her CV was rammed full of experience. It just also showed so many moves and three maternity breaks as she juggled with her children's needs and her husband's constant moving around to "get ahead". All very well for him to say that there are schools everywhere don't worry, but no one wanted a teacher who had a habit of moving on after a couple of years. Nor did they appreciate one who kept popping out children. Even if they would all be out of business if no one did. She had had seven interviews before she landed this job. Each Head Teacher had said the same thing. "You are an excellent teacher and you interviewed very well. However, we went with someone else this time." Each time a younger, fresher version of Katie had been the chosen one. This school had been the last in a reasonable radius from home. It had been her last chance to go back to work now her youngest was at school and she had grabbed it with both hands. Never mind it was Mondays and Fridays, the worst two days in a week and in foundation stage, she would adapt.

Joan could see a school. A vision of her little granddaughter in her new school uniform swam into her mind. Lucy! Lucy will know where her mother is. She walked up to the school gate. It was locked. She waited.

"Lucy, it's your turn to read."
Lucy looked down at the activity on the table in front of her. She just needed to find a number six then she would have them all in a row- 1-10 and she could tell Mummy what she had done.
"Lucy come on now get your book!" Still Lucy stayed starring at the blocks. The teacher was standing over her now.
"Lucy didn't you hear me? Am I going to have to put your name on the stop sign?" Lucy felt sick. Mummy didn't like it when her name was on the stop sign. She got all excited when it was on the sunshine sign, which didn't happen very often. Lucy tried her best but when she was doing something good like sticking these blocks together no one ever noticed.
"Lucy! Get your book!"
Lucy jumped at the anger in the teacher's voice then stumbled across to her tray. She fished out her book and went to stand by the teacher. There it was. Her name L-u-c-y spelled out on the stop sign. She opened the book and tried to read but the letters got all muddled as her tummy hurt and she couldn't remember them.
"g-o…"

"Yes... "
"Go?"
"Yes, go on."
"Go on? "Repeated Lucy.
"No look at the letters Lucy! T-o doesn't make on." Lucy looked bewildered. Why had the teacher said, "go on," if it wasn't go on? The teacher wrote something in her reading record. Somehow, she knew Mummy wouldn't like it.

Slowly other people started to arrive at the school gates. Joan smiled at them all benignly. They stood in little groups and chatted. Some of them looked at Joan curiously yet no one spoke to her. A few turned away quickly when they saw her looking at them. There were whispers. Finally, the gate opened and the mothers surged through. Joan went with them. They stood in the playground and waited as one by one children in blue uniforms came out of the school to meet their parents. Joan watched the last child go through the gate. Where was Lucy? She walked into the school. She must still be inside. The foyer was full of pretty pictures. Had Lucy drawn any? She stopped to admire them.

"Excuse me who are you?" Joan jumped. She turned to see a tall, stern looking woman peering at her through a Perspex window.

"I'm Lucy's Grandma, Joan Jessup." Joan smiled at the woman.

"Oh, have you come to collect her?"

"Yes."

"What class is she in?" Joan frowned.

"Katie's, she's a teacher you know."

"Wait here." The woman picked up her phone and pressed some numbers. Joan couldn't hear what she was saying. She was cold. There was a radiator and a comfortable chair. She sat down and held her hands to the radiator rubbing them vigorously together.

Katie was finished for the day. At least she had finished teaching. She was tidying the classroom, so the job share had nothing to complain about. Then she would sit and mark her books so all would be ready for the next day. At least there was very little to mark in foundation. She took out her bag to find her favourite green pen. Her phone was on top where she had shoved it earlier. Six missed calls. Four were from Jack! He had also sent four texts all asking in increasingly impolite terms where she was. She shrugged off her frustration at his inability to remember her working days and rang him back.

"Hi Jack, what's up?"

"I've been trying to reach you all day, this project is dragging on and on…" She put the phone within hearing distance and picked up her pen to start marking.

Lucy bounced into after school club. At last, the learning stuff was over and she could play. She pulled on a witch's costume and started to stir an imaginary cauldron full of spells…

"I think perhaps you have the wrong school."

A new lady was smiling at Joan, although she wasn't making any sense. "We don't have another Katie teaching here, only me."

"But you're not my daughter!"

"No… we are a bit concerned about your granddaughter. Were you here to pick her up?"

"Yes. Yes, I told the other lady, Lucy Jessup!"

"We don't have a Lucy Jessup in this school. Perhaps she goes to a different one?" Joan looked around her. If Lucy wasn't here, then where was she? And Katie, it was Katie she needed. Katie would know what to do. Where was Katie?

"I need Katie."

The kind lady smiled, "I'll help you find her. Wait here."

Joan sat back down. The radiator had gone off and the room was getting cold. She thought of her warm home. She knew she had come here for a reason, yet it didn't seem important now. The kind lady was gone. There was just the fierce looking one watching her. She shifted uncomfortably in her chair. The dog would be hungry. What time was it? She was hungry. She had better go home.

She headed to the door. The kind lady touched her arm.

"No don't go please, I'll find Katie."
"I want to go home."
"Where do you live Joan?"
"Home…"
"Come back inside and have a cup of tea. Tell me more about Lucy."

"So anyway, I won't be home in time to pick up Matt tonight." Katie grabbed the phone.
"What!"
"I have to work late and can't pick up our son."
"We agreed! You pick him up after football because I have to get Lucy and Molly from after school club and I can't be in two places at one time."
"You will have to call the school then and tell them."
"Tell them what?"
"That you will be late I guess."
Furious, Katie snatched up her bag and ran for the door. If she was quick, she could grab the girls and get across town to Matt before the boys were all finished changing. The PE teacher would still be around so Matt wouldn't be abandoned. Now he was in secondary school teachers were less careful to ensure they went home with a parent. Matt wasn't ready for managing busses yet.

Lucy's face was contorted with rage. She had been flying her broomstick around the room with gleeful abandon and now Mummy was all cross and wanted her to hurry as they had to go in the car. She stamped her little foot.
"I don't want to!"
Perfect Molly had fetched her coat and bags, "Come on Lucy we need to help Mum." Lucy stuck out her tongue at her sister.

"So, Lucy wears a red uniform?"
"Yes, yes, it is very bright. She looked so smart on her first day. Katie took pictures. I have one next to the one of Molly and Matt."
"You have more grandchildren? How lovely. Excuse me a second."

The kind lady hissed to the stern one. "I think the granddaughter is at St John's. Foundation at a guess. And she has a brother and sister- Molly and Matt."

"I've rung every school in the area looking for a Lucy Jessup. The old lady is clearly losing her marbles. She's not my responsibility and I need to go home."

"I think the children may have a different surname, after all her daughter is probably married if she has three kids. Please just try St John's and see if they have three children with those names." Katy Bishop was a newly qualified teacher. She had been amazed to land the role in year three as the other interviewee had been so much more experienced. She couldn't leave this bewildered old lady to walk home in her slippers. Although she was a little afraid of the secretary who ran the school with firm efficiency.

Katie's phone was ringing again and again. She wished she had shut it off. She was driving as fast as she dared. A sullen, sulky Lucy was strapped in the back next to her increasingly quiet middle child. Molly had become rather too perfect recently…

Matt was waiting at the gate. He looked tired and cross. Wordlessly he threw his kit into the boot and climbed in next to Katie.

"Have you got any food?"

"No, I've come straight from work." Snarling he sunk down in his seat. The phone buzzed. This time she reluctantly answered.

"Is that Katie Robinson?"

"Yes."

"This is Katy Bishop from Garrett's Hall school. I believe we have your mother here, Joan Jessup?"

"That's my mum. Why is she there?"

"She came in looking for your daughter Lucy. She seems very confused. Can you come and get her."

Katie glanced at her children. It would be another half hour in the car to get her mother and take her home. To say nothing of the time it would take to settle her down before she could leave her. At least she could fix the food problem. There was a pizza place next to Grandma's.

"I'm on my way."

Joan was comfortable at last. Katie had been and all the children. She had brought pizza for tea. And she had stuck a big sign on her door to remind her to take her keys next time she went out. Katie was wonderful.

Lucy was snuggled up to Mummy in her bed. Mummy was reading her a story. They hadn't done the dreaded reading book as it was so late and she was tired. No one had mentioned stop signs and she had had pizza for dinner. She smiled happily as she drifted off to sleep.

Katie loaded Matt's kit into the washing machine and tidied the kitchen. She had made Jack a meal for when he came home. The children were all asleep. She felt bone weary. She was going to have to do something about her mum, although she didn't know what. Thank goodness for that lovely young teacher though. Now where had she seen her before…

Two weeks later, nothing had changed and mornings remained the worst time of day.

"C'mon Matt we need to get going."

Matt shovelled his last mouthful of cereal into his mouth before grabbing his bag and joining a frustrated Katie at the door.

"You didn't brush your teeth."

"No time," said Matt spitting bits of half chewed cereal from the sides of his mouth. Katie knew she should remind him of his manners and send him to brush his teeth, but if she was to have any chance of getting to school on time she needed to leave right now. Molly and Lucy were miraculously already in the car. She managed a half-hearted, "don't speak with your mouth full and be quicker next time as you don't want cavities," while she ushered her son out of the door. As she started down the drive her phone rang. She saw her mother's number flash up. She quickly pressed ignore and carried on down the drive. She was sure it would be nothing important.

Joan stared at her phone. Why had it gone dead like that? Should she try again? She pressed the numbers carefully to be sure she had Katie's number right. It started to ring. It carried on ringing. No one picked it up. How odd. Katie always answered. She had one of those mobile phones she could take everywhere. She shook her head and wandered into the living room. She only wanted to know what she was doing today. Katie always knew. She hoped it was lunch day. She loved it when Katie took her for lunch at the garden centre. That was on a Wednesday usually. Was it Wednesday?

Thankfully the phone didn't ring again and Katie got Matt and the girls dropped off at their respective schools before turning to cross the town to get to hers. It was a tricky drive in the rush hour even with the back route she had found. While she had to go over a few speed bumps, it was better than the main road which went at a snail's pace. At least it was if there weren't too many people pressing the pedestrian crossing lights. It drove her crazy when people pressed the button then crossed without waiting for the lights as the road was clear. She would then have to sit at the lights while no one crossed. Worse than that this morning a group of school children on bikes pressed the button as they rode by with no intention at all of crossing. She glared at their retreating backs as she sat waiting for the lights to change. Her phone rang again - Mum. She never answered the phone when driving. Absolutely never. It was the third call and she was stuck waiting. She grabbed it.
    "I only have a second Mum is there a problem?"
    "Um well is it lunch day?"
    "Huh?"
    "Are we having lunch?" The lights changed. It was a slow road. Katie stuck the phone under her chin precariously.
    "No Mum I am going to work. I have to go now." She dropped the phone without switching it off. She could hear her mum.
    "Kate? Katie? What day is it then?" She pulled over.

"It's Monday Mum. I'm on my way to work. Can't come over today Sorry. Why don't you take Trixie for a nice walk? It looks like it will be warm."

"Yes, I could do that. Can't you come for lunch then?"

"No Mum I'm working."

"Oh Ok."

"I have to go."

"See you later then."

"Bye Mum."

"Just a minute. What day is it?" Too late, Katie had switched off the phone and was pulling back out into the traffic.

Joan put the phone back in its holder. Katie wasn't coming. So, what should she do? She went back into the living room and turned on the TV. The screen was blank. She pressed various buttons on the remote. Nothing. She would have to ring Katie. She shuffled back out to the hall.

Katie had squeezed her car into the last available space in the school car park and was running for the door as her phone went off again. She stopped and glanced at the screen. Mum again! She had no time to deal with this. Tomorrow she would visit her mum and make sure she had a good day. Today was work. She pressed ignore and turned the phone to silent. Taking a deep breath and slowing to a walk she went through into reception.

Joan starred at the phone. Why wasn't Katie there? Her phone must be faulty. She sighed and looked back at her blank TV. No Katie, no phone and no TV. What should she do? At that moment Trixie came up wagging her tail hopefully.

"Come on then. Let's find your lead." The little dog's tail wagged furiously as Joan clipped on her lead, put on her coat and headed for the door. As she opened it, she saw Katie's big bright sign reminding her to take her keys.

"I have them already!" she said out loud as she swallowed down the knot of sadness. "Where was Katie and why wouldn't she come?"

Chapter 2

Changes

"Katie, can I have a minute please?"

Katie knew that tone. Deputy heads always used it when something was up. Otherwise, it would be a quick chat in the staffroom. Now what on earth had she done? She followed Jill into her office.

"Do take a seat." Why did her palms feel sweaty, just like a naughty child being told off? What could she have done?

"Don't look so worried it isn't a major issue." Uh oh so it was an issue.

"It's just about your late arrivals in the morning. You don't seem to be getting in much before registration."

"That was agreed," blurted Katie. "I asked for that at my interview as I have to get my children to school; two different schools."

"I appreciate that and we have understood until now. However, it has been a while and other staff are starting to murmur about it. You aren't the only parent on the staff you know." Jill smiled. It reminded Katie of a tiger about to eat its prey.

"I understand your oldest is at secondary school now. Perhaps it is time for him to start using the bus. A bit of independence wouldn't hurt. And the little one has had almost a month to get used to school so maybe now she could go to breakfast club." She had it all worked out. Katie's mind wavered between how dare you interfere in my family life to yes it would make my life easier to not have to do the mad school run before I get here. All that came out of her mouth was:

"I will have to look into it and see if breakfast club has any spaces. I have two daughters to think of. And check bus times."

"I'm sure you will be able to sort it out. So 8am start for you next week please. Staff briefings are prompt at 8am each day." Katie smiled weakly and left the room.

Joan was feeling lonely. She had taken the dog for its walk but wasn't sure what to do next. Was there somewhere she needed to go? She couldn't think what day it was. She would need to ask Katie. She went to the telephone. Next to it was Katie's notice. In big letters, it said:

Katie's number is 07654 234362.

Katie is at work on Mondays and Fridays.

Joan frowned. Was it Monday? Or even Friday? She needed to ring Katie to ask. She looked at the number again. What if she was at work? She knew she mustn't ring when Katie was at work. She went to her calendar, but she hadn't remembered to tick off the days. Or had she? She turned on the TV, perhaps they would say the day? A gardening show was on. She liked that presenter. She sat down to watch.

Lucy was doing number sentences in her book. She loved numbers. They made more sense than letters and there weren't so many to remember. At least she kind of knew there were more but they were all just the same ones put together and that made sense. They always sounded the same too. Not like silly letters that just got jumbled. She happily filled in the answers, smiling as she wrote them down. The teacher called her name.

"Lucy!" Lucy didn't like it when the teacher stopped her, but she knew she had to put her pencil down and look at the teacher.

"Can you bring me your book please?" That was OK she had done lots of work. Proudly she took her book to the teacher's desk.

"Show me what you have done Lucy." Lucy pointed to the rows of numbers. The teacher looked. She frowned.

"That one is wrong." She said pointing to the third sum. You have written a 6 when it should have been a 9. Lucy's happy smile faded. She had done so many. Why would the teacher only look at the one that was wrong? The teacher wrote something on a piece of paper.

"Put this in your book bag for your mum later please Lucy."

Lucy took the paper and slowly went to her tray and shoved it in. No way was she putting that in her bag tonight. Why did the teacher only ever notice what she did wrong! Biting her lip with disappointment she went back to her seat. The numbers all looked blurry now and she couldn't concentrate.

The gardening programme had ended. Joan got up. She needed to go somewhere although she wasn't sure where. She wanted to ask Katie, but the paper said not to ring. Not on Mondays or Fridays. How would she know if it was one of those days if she couldn't ask Katie? At least she shouldn't ring. Maybe she could just pop into the school? She put on her coat and shoes and headed to the door. TAKE YOUR KEYS said the sign on the door. She picked them up off the hook and carefully locked the door behind her. She set off down the street.

The secretary heard the doorbell. She tried to see who it was, but they were standing too far back. She buzzed them in. Probably just a delivery. She sighed when she saw the old lady shuffle in.

"Your grandchildren aren't at this school." She said firmly.

"I, I wasn't looking for them? Am I supposed to be picking them up?" Joan stumbled over her words.

"I don't know what you are meant to be doing, they aren't here."

"I, I was looking for Katie?"

"Your Katie?"

"Well yes of course my Katie."

"She's not here either. You have the wrong school. Again."

"Sorry…my mistake."

Joan turned to go.

"Mrs Jessup! Is that you!" Joan turned to see a smiling face she vaguely recognised.

"Did you come to see me. How lovely! I have a few minutes between classes. Come and sit in reception and let's have a chat."

Katy Bishop shot a glance at the disapproving secretary as she took Joan's arm and led her to a comfy seat.

"So, what are you up to today?"

Matt was hungry as always and devouring his food. Molly ate daintily and Lucy was uncharacteristically quiet. Katie tried to pick her moment carefully. She had read the timetables at lunchtime and had to admit a bus journey wasn't too difficult for Matt.

"Matt?" He glanced up, still shovelling food into his overstuffed mouth.

Katie stopped herself from commenting on his poor table manners and focussed on the matter at hand.

"I was wondering if you could take the bus to school on my workdays from next week. I've looked at the times and I think it could work. You…"

"Really! Wow Mum that'd be great!" Gravy oozed from one corner of his mouth as he grinned with delight.

"You don't mind?"

"Mind? I get out of being stuck with these two in the car for ages. I get to ride with my mates. What's not to like? Can I do it every day?"

"Um…well… let's start with two days and see shall we." Matt shrugged and went back to his food.

While Molly accepted the idea of breakfast club readily enough, Lucy was a different matter. She burst into tears and ran from the room. Katie was confused. Lucy loved after school club and it was the same people who ran breakfast club. She left her own dinner to grow cold and went to find her youngest.

"So why don't you want to go to breakfast club sweetheart?" Lucy scrunched up her face and refused to answer.

"Your best friend Charlotte goes. You could play together."

"She's not my best friend anymore."

"Oh, why's that."

"Because Jojo is."

"Oh OK. Does Jojo go to breakfast club?"

"Yes."

"So, you could play with her then." Lucy frowned. Mummy hadn't really understood. It wasn't her friends who were the problem. It was school. School was horrible. Then again, Mummy was offering her ice cream for pudding if she went back and finished dinner. Reluctantly she wiped her eyes.

Joan had had a nice day. That lovely young Katy who wasn't her Katie had told her about a little coffee shop where people went to drink coffee and chat. She had been there for a few hours and talked to lots of nice people. She wasn't sure she could remember their names, although she would remember Katy Bishop. She reminded her of her Katie when she was younger. She always had time for her mother then. Katie had been tired on the phone that evening. She hadn't rung while Katie was at school, although that didn't seem to help. Katie was still grumpy and short with her. Something about a long day. Never mind, tomorrow was Tuesday. She could ring any time on Tuesday.

Next morning Lucy was trying to hide under her covers. She didn't want to go to school. She hadn't taken the note home and now she thought the teacher would be even crosser. And then Mummy would be cross. She had tried so hard and she didn't mean to get one sum wrong.
"Come on Lucy we have to have breakfast!"
Katie felt Lucy's forehead. It was not hot. She did look a bit pale. Katie needed today after working Monday. Tuesday was cleaning day. The big post weekend clear up always got delayed to Tuesday now she worked Mondays.
"Come on sweetheart let's give today a chance. I'll let your teacher know that you don't feel too brilliant and she can call me lunchtime if needs be to collect you."
Reluctantly Lucy got out of bed. Slowly she dressed and brushed her teeth. She walked as slowly as she could to the car.
"Come ON Lucy!" yelled Matt. "See Mum, I should get the bus every day!" Katie's phone rang.
"Not now Mum, I'm just taking the children to school…."
"I just need to know…"
"I'll call you back in an hour, I promise."

"… what day it is?" Katie had hung up.

Katie held Lucy's hand firmly as they walked through the school gates. The class teacher smiled as she approached her.

"Mrs Robinson, so you got my note!"

"Er no, I was just going to tell you Lucy wasn't keen to come today. She doesn't seem ill, just unhappy…did she do something wrong?"

"Far from it! I wanted to ask you if she could join my extra numbers club. I hold it after school on a Wednesday. It's for children who show real promise in maths. Lucy does, she did some excellent work yesterday, far above average for her age. We play lots of games that involve counting. We do puzzles and build with various construction toys. It's not formal learning but it helps develop those skills."

"What do you think Lucy? Would you like to stay after school on Wednesdays and play numbers games?"

Lucy looked from the teacher to her mummy. So, no one was cross? It didn't matter that she got one wrong? The note had been a Good Thing? And now she was going to get to do extra games?" She nodded sheepishly.

"Excellent!" said her teacher, "We will expect you tomorrow." She smiled as Lucy took her bags from her mummy and skipped off into class. Katie turned to go. There was something she needed to do. Oh yes ring Mum. She reached for her phone.

"Hey Mum what's up?"

Chapter 3

Katy Bishop

October 2018

Katy Bishop loved her job. In filling her days with productive hours helping young minds flourish, she replenished her void both practically and emotionally. At least that worked during school hours. If she was lucky, she could spend much of the evening marking or preparing lessons. Then her tiny flat needed cleaning, her clothes washing and ironing, so she always looked immaculate for work. What was it Julian had sneered? Teachers are always so dowdy. Her reflex to his criticism was to make a point of being smart with bright, fashionable but still sensible clothes. It wasn't easy on a budget, although she had plenty of time at the weekends to browse charity shops and discount stores. She got lots of lovely stationery from those too. There was nothing quite a like a new set of highlighters. If her mind wandered and whispered of loneliness, she simply focussed harder on one of her young charges' needs. And she never, ever, looked backwards.

Joan Jessup had wandered into her life in a random moment. Katy's instinctive reaction to the old lady's plight had been to help. That first cup of tea and pointing her to the friendly café gatherings had been enough. Yet she found herself drawn to Joan. Did loneliness seek out friends?

"Hello?" Joan looked confused.

"It's Katy!"

Joan shook her head. "You're not Katie!"

Katy smiled, "Sorry I forgot your daughter's name is Katie too isn't it. I'm the other Katy; from the school across the road. You've been to see us a few times."

A broad smile swept Joan's face. "Oh yes, I know now. How lovely to see you. Do come in."

And so began a Friday afternoon ritual. Katy would pack up straight after the children left, leaving her marking for home. Then she would cross the road and pop in on Joan. They would have tea and biscuits and chat about anything. Joan would tell the same few stories of her childhood or of Katie as a child and occasionally her late husband. However, mostly she liked to hear about Katy's day. She loved to hear stories of the children she taught and would often punctuate Katy's tales with, "Oh my Lucy would say that," or "My Matt would have enjoyed that lesson". Her world seemed very small, even smaller than Katy's. Somehow that comforted Katy.

As time passed Katy began to do occasional little jobs with Joan. It started with pruning the roses in front of her house. Joan was struggling to break the dead heads off with her hands when Katy arrived. Seeing the tiny cuts and scratches on the old lady's arms Katy whipped out her sharpest scissors from her briefcase and gently took over. Joan gratefully conceded and then disappeared inside. She emerged ten minutes later with a proper set of secateurs and spent a delightful half an hour giving Katy a lesson in how roses should be pruned. For all her forgetfulness some things seemed to remain. Her garden looked like a wasteland now but obviously she had once known how to tend it. That inspired Katy to pull out her favourite highlighters and create a little gardening rota for Joan. A job to do each day. They searched out all her tools and made careful note on the chart of where they were. A little help with organisation and Joan was able to reconnect to an activity she loved. And another moment of satisfaction for Katy.

"Now Katy love, tell me a bit about you?"

Their weekly ritual usually began this way and Katy would set off with the latest school story.

"Well today Emma…"

"Maybe not about school this time. How about family? Or do you have a young man?"

Katy stared at the kindly face she had used to hide her tragedies behind. Her mouth opened and closed but only silence came out.

"Oh dear. Have I said something wrong? Tell me about-Emma was it?"

Katy forced a smile. "It's OK. I just don't talk about my parents much. They died. Both of them. Car accident. Two years ago." The staccato sentences left her breathless. But she needed to say it all. All of it, just once. Then maybe she could breathe out. "My boyfriend was driving. He'd been drinking. He wasn't kind. He used to bully me. I don't know why I let him. He left afterwards. Said he couldn't stand my endless moping. I went back to university and got my teacher's certificate. And moved away. Gave me something positive to do. You know. Help people."

Two big tears coursed down the old lady's wrinkled cheeks. Wordlessly she reached over and put her arms around Katy. She stroked her back and made soothing noises. They stayed like that for a long pause and then Joan stood up.

"I'll pop the kettle on. Make another cup of tea."

Chapter 4

Shopping

November 2018

"Katie where are you?" Jack's exasperated voice rang through the whole house.

"I'm just helping Lucy with her uniform. What's the matter?" Katie tried hard to keep her frustration out of her voice.

"There's no jam."

Sighing, Katie pulled Lucy's pinafore over her head rather too roughly, eliciting a squeal from her daughter.

"Sorry sweetheart, can you manage your socks yourself I have to help Daddy," she muttered as she rushed down the stairs.

Smiling she opened the spares cupboard; the one that was always stocked with tins and jars. Then anything essential - like Jack's favourite jam – was always available.

"Don't worry there's…" she started but he cut her off sharply.

"I'm not stupid, I looked in there. You have let it all run down."

Jack was right, the cupboard was short of so many things. She knew she needed to do a big shop. Lately she had been taking her mother with her on her weekly shop so she could make sure she had some healthy foods in too. Her mother seemed to only have ice cream and chocolate in if she didn't. Shopping with her mum was such hard work as she seemed to struggle to make any decisions. The number of times she would turn to Katie and say, "do I like that?" It all took twice as long.

"I'll do a big shop today, after I've popped in on Mum." Jack who was making a show of spreading marmalade thinly on his toast paused and stared straight at his wife.

"Perhaps you should prioritise the shopping today."

Katie took a deep breath and forced a smile. "I think I can manage both and I didn't see Mum yesterday as I was at work."

"Oh yes, how could I forget." Katie winced at the barely disguised sarcasm.

"Oh, I know it is important to you. And your mother is important to you and the children's activities are important to you. I just wonder if I am at all important to you." Jack got up leaving his toast uneaten, carefully folded his newspaper and slotted it into his briefcase as Katie stared open mouthed at him.

"I need you to pick up my dry cleaning today if it's not too much trouble. I have a major presentation tomorrow and need my grey suit." He left before Katie could frame any kind of response.

Joan was sitting waiting by the front window when Katie arrived. A broad smile lit up her face when she saw her daughter. She walked to the door but as always it was locked. Frowning, she turned back to the kitchen to find her keys. After a frantic search in cupboards, drawers and her handbag she finally located them and shuffled to the door to let Katie in.

"I think we need to put a hook somewhere to hang your keys," said Katie for the umpteenth time.

"Oh, it's no problem I just forgot where I put them today," replied her mother cheerfully as if it were an unusual occurrence.

"At least I don't forget them when I leave." She smiled indicating the large sign Katie had stuck on the door saying, "Take your keys," after the time Joan had shut herself out.

"Where are we going today?"

"Well, I thought we could just have a cuppa. I need to get a few things done today."

"Like what?"

"Well," she hesitated, knowing what her mother's response would be, "I have to do a big shop and go to the dry cleaners." Then mop the floors, scrub the bathroom and catch up on the ironing she thought inwardly.

"Why don't I come too! I can help pack the bags and maybe I need a few bits myself." Joan smiled brightly.

"Do you, I thought we stocked your fridge last time we shopped...let's check."

Katie opened the fridge. The vegetable crisper was full of the wilting, healthy vegetables she had crammed it with last week. The yoghurts were all out of date and unopened. A piece of uncooked fish competed with a ready cooked piece of chicken for the least appetising, longest ignored item. Cheese, bread and eggs sat on the top shelf while the door held a pint of milk, a half-drunk bottle of wine and the tell-tale large bar of chocolate, half eaten. The freezer was still full of easy microwave dinners. With two tubs of fancy ice creams and a packet of Magnums.

"Oh, Mum you haven't had any of your vegetables. What did you have for dinner last night?"

"I just fancied some scrambled eggs. Not much point cooking when it's only for me." Katie glanced at the fruit bowl. Still full of over-ripe fruit. Only the bananas were gone. In the cupboard were the tins of soup and beans she had picked out for her mother as easy healthy choices. The cakes and biscuits were all gone. She forced herself to smile.

"I guess you had better come with me then. First, we need to throw out some of this out-of-date stuff. We can't have you getting food poisoning." Half an hour later, after scrubbing off the mould lurking in the back of the fridge Katie and Joan left for the supermarket.

All the way there Joan kept up a running commentary on the people and places they passed. That man is always waiting for the bus, we went to that shop once for a bar of soap, we walked down that path by the river and fed the ducks, that lady has too many bags to carry every day. None of it seemed to make any sense to Katie. Why would her mum go all this way just for soap? And they never went to the shops at the same time for that man to always be at the stop. Joan rattled on cheerfully enough and at least it allowed Katie to think about Jack's behaviour as her mother's monologue didn't seem to need any responses from her.

She was used to Jack being self-centred. He was an only child with an overindulgent mother. Katie had worked hard over the years to help him see a little beyond his own needs. Lately he had been sharp with her too often and was snapping at the children over little things: too much noise, toys in the living room, dirty shoes in the hall. Things she usually dealt with before he got home, she realised. That was the problem. She had learned to keep the peace by keeping the chaos of children out of his sight. Since she had returned to work, she had had less time to mop up all their debris. Even so he should not be treating her like that. She resolved to speak to him about it again. Gently nudge him into understanding the pressure she was under. He ought to help her a little more now. As should the children. The older two at least could be a bit more responsible. She would do a big shop, sort the house out, cook his favourite meal and then bring it up. Once she had shown she was still on top of things. Feeling strengthened by her resolve she turned her attention back to Joan.

"That poor dog, that man walks him too much. Every day he is going up and down this road."

"So, have you thought about what you need to buy Mum? Do you need any dog food?"

"Oh, I'll just see what I fancy when I get in there."

"Ok… I need rather a lot today so maybe we can go around separately with a trolley each."

"That's no fun. We can't chat while we shop then. I can help you find what you need if we stick together. I don't need much, I'm sure it can all fit in one trolley." Katie looked at her mums forced bright smile with the worry lurking in her eyes and realised this trip was going to be just the same as the rest. At least she must make sure she bought at least three jars of jam!

Two hours later they emerged from the shop. The trolley was piled high with everything Katie could grab while trying to steer her mother through the crowded aisles. She had long abandoned her list as Joan had stood vacantly time and again staring at the rows of food. "Do I like salmon? Or would tuna be better? Does this keep? I need more eggs. I think I'll have scrambled eggs tonight. Where are the eggs? I need some ice cream." Katie decided to let her mother pile up her own choices. What was the point in more wasted food. Yet the three packets of biscuits, two lots of jam tarts and five packets of cakes appalled her. Why on earth was her mother suddenly eating like this? Her mum had always been so particular about vegetables and fruit when she was growing up. As they neared the till the answer dawned on her. Perhaps her mum was having difficulties cooking. Maybe she needed to try a different tack.

"How about some salad Mum? Do you think you would like some tomatoes with your eggs tonight?"

"Oooh what a lovely idea! Where do we find those?" Katie sighed as she realised the salad was right back at the other end of the supermarket. As they worked their way back against the tide, she also slipped some fruit juices into her mum's selections. At least she can wash down her cakes with some vitamins!

By the time Katie had taken Joan home and unpacked her shopping, made her a cup of tea and a sandwich laden with salad it was close to school pick up time. She couldn't believe how the day had vanished. She rushed home and practically threw her own multitude of shopping into her cupboards while munching a cookie and a banana to stave off her own hunger pangs. She liked to walk home with the younger children when she could even though that meant leaving early to walk there. It seemed a bit pointless when she then had to pile them in the car to drive to Matt's school, yet the half an hour or so chatting as they ambled home gave her a good chance to catch up with her girls' day. With just 15 minutes to get there she was going to have to run. Lucy didn't like it when she was the last mum through the gate.

Two hours later Katie was feeling accomplished. The children had all completed their homework and had agreed to tidy up their toys into their own rooms. They had been cooperative, even enthusiastic about helping with some chores, especially when the offer of ice cream for dessert was mentioned. Katie had somehow managed to slip one of Joan's tubs into her bag as she knew her mum's freezer had no more space. The tough jobs like mopping the floor had to wait, although even Lucy had enjoyed some dusting and the whole house looked fresher. She had taken a little extra trouble with dinner. Jack's favourite roast chicken, Matt's crispy roast potatoes, Molly's mashed swede and Lucy's carrots. Then ice cream for dessert. She smiled as she set the table putting a fresh vase of daffodils in the centre. This was going to be a nice family meal.

Jack crashed through the door, laden with briefcase and extra files. She went to greet him with a smile and a kiss. He brushed her cheek perfunctorily.

"Did you pick up my suit…"

Chapter 5

Christmas is Coming!

December 2018

"Mummy! Look I want one of those for Christmas?" Lucy was pointing at the screen and yelling. Katie swivelled round eager to see her daughter's latest wish. Christmas shopping was becoming urgent yet so far, she had only managed the inevitable new Arsenal football kit for Matt.

"But you already have a dolls house sweetheart."

"Yes, but Mummy that one has little animals in it- see!"

"Couldn't you just put animals in the one you have?" She was rewarded with a pout.

"Well yesterday you wanted a Barbie car. Why don't you sit down a write a letter to Santa then he will know what you want most of all."

Lucy considered this carefully, writing was not her favourite activity, but she did need Santa to know.

"I'll just tell you Mummy. Then you can tell Santa. Matt says that's what you do anyway." Katie was aware Matt and probably Molly no longer believed, but she was grateful he hadn't spoiled it for his little sister. The magic of Christmas could prevail a little longer.

"OK sweetheart you need to tell me soon. Santa is very busy this time of year." At that moment Molly wandered in. Katie decided to ask her what she was hoping for.

"We were talking about Christmas Molly. Do you have any wishes?"

"I want an animal house and a Barbie car!" chipped in Lucy, "Oh and one of those!" Like most parents Katie hated TV adverts at this time of year.

Molly shook her head gently.

"There must be something you would like. What about some new art supplies? Or a pretty dress? "

"I can't have what I want so it doesn't matter."

"What is it you want Molly? If you don't tell me, I can't help."

"Mum's going to phone Santa, so he knows so you need to tell her!"

"Thanks Lucy. Now come in the kitchen with me Molly, away from the TV and we can talk properly." Molly followed dutifully into the kitchen and sat down. Katie poured her a glass of milk and grabbed the biscuit jar. She sat down opposite and smiled at her daughter.

"So, what is it?"

Molly shook her head again.

"Come on Molls tell me. Even if you can't have it, we could at least consider it together and work out why."

"I know why."

"OK, so tell me."

Molly looked up her big eyes wide and sad, "I'd like a pet of my own. But I know I can't because Dad is allergic to fur."

"Oh Molly. We have had this conversation before. You are right we can't have pets in the house because of Dad's allergy. He can't help it you know."

"I know."

"Why do you want it so badly?"

Molly looked down at her hands. "I…well…Matt doesn't play with me anymore now he's so old. And Lucy is OK, but she plays little girl games. I can't go to a friend's houses after school so much now you work. And you are with Grandma lots. It would be nice to have a puppy or kitten to play with. Or even a hamster. They don't have much fur."

Katie sighed, "I'm sorry sweetheart your dad is adamant no pets allowed. Not even very small ones. You know he can't set foot in Grandma's house without sneezing, even if she puts Trixie outside."

"I know. But that's what I wanted. Anyway, some art stuff will be nice. That's OK." The look in her eyes showed clearly it was not OK. Katie tried another tack.

"How about I take you over to Grandma's with me a bit more often, at least at the weekends. I don't think Grandma can walk so far these days. You can take Trixie for a lovely walk on your own. Would you like that? No crossing busy roads mind you, but you can get to the little copse Grandma goes to just walking straight down the road. What do you think?"

"That would be nice. Thanks Mummy." Molly's little smile didn't quite reach her eyes.

Later that evening Katie decided to broach the issue with Jack. She really couldn't see how a hamster could set off his allergies. Not if it lived in Molly's room. He rarely set foot in there and if he couldn't anymore perhaps the benefit to Molly would be worth it. Or even worth a few sneezes on his part.

"I've been talking to the children about Christmas presents today."

"Hmmm."

"What they would like."

"Well go ahead and get it then; just don't spend above our limit." Jack had clearly defined limits for Christmas spending that Katie adhered to carefully by bargain hunting and syphoning a little off the weekly shopping bill for the months leading up to it. They could afford to splash out a little, but Jack believed children shouldn't be spoilt and budgeted accordingly. Katie agreed in principle although she didn't think Jack really understood the cost of children's toys let alone football kits! A hamster, even with a good quality cage would be below budget.

"Yes of course. In fact, Molly doesn't want anything too big. Very small actually."

"Good."

"Jack- I need you to focus on this!"

Jack pulled his eyes away from the TV screen.

"Why?"

Katie bit her lip and began carefully.

"Molly is feeling a bit lonely lately. Matt is obsessed with football and Lucy is so much younger. She would like to have something of her own to play with."

"She has tons of toys!"

"Yes…not a toy…something alive."

"What!"

"A pet…just a small one in her room…like a hamster."

"Katie I cannot have pets in the house I am allergic to fur. You know that."

"I do…but she was so sad about it. And she could keep it in her room all the time. You wouldn't have to go in there at all."

"So I am to be banished from my daughter's room in favour of a rodent!"

"No…well yes sort of…but you don't often go in there."

"Hardly the point is it. And as you well know if she has been handling it and comes out of her room, she brings the problem with her."

"I would tell her to wash her hands every time."

"What if the thing escaped?"

"I'll buy a good cage."

"She's a child she might leave the door open."

"Oh Jack you are being silly now. Molly is very responsible."

"Silly! Me! I think perhaps you are the one who is being silly! I have a very severe allergy to all forms of fur and you want to bring a furry creature into my house. What's more you have given our daughter hope that you might so she will be upset when you say no…"

"I haven't! I said no. I just thought I would ask you anyway."

"That's OK then. The answer remains no and you will have to find something else that she wants."

Jack picked up the remote and changed channels to the news.

Later as they were getting ready for bed Jack unexpectedly returned to the subject.

"I am sorry you know."

"For what?"

"That I can't let Molly have a pet. I know how much she would like one. But what if we agreed and then I was ill because of it and we had to get rid of it? That would be far worse. I just thought you had given her hope…and that wouldn't be fair."

Katie sighed and looked squarely at her husband. She really didn't think a little hamster in Molly's room would make him ill, but he clearly did. And equally clearly, he did have Molly's best interests at heart. At least she decided she would give him the benefit of the doubt.

"It's OK love she understands. I will get her something else really special. I just can't think what at the moment. And as for Lucy she wants everything."

"Hmm I'm sure you will make a good decision."

Jack had moved on.

The next morning Katie sat at her computer searching online. She found some bright new acrylic paints for Molly along with some real canvasses. Molly had never been allowed acrylics before as they didn't wash out easily, so Katie reasoned it would make her feel more grown up. She also looked at some sequin art kits and oil painting by numbers. She decided to add a sparkling sequin kit of three penguins. As she was browsing, she saw an advert from a photography studio offering cut price family portraits in the run up to Christmas. The last professional photos she had of her family were from way back when Lucy was a baby. On impulse she phoned and booked an appointment for the following Saturday. That could be her Christmas present to herself! One of the perks of going back to work she realised, was she could splash out a little extra. She went back to Molly's order and added an oil set after all.

Chapter 6

Photo Shoot

December 2018

Joan was sitting in her chair. She thought Katie would be arriving soon although she really wasn't sure. It was Saturday. She knew that as she had bought herself a paper. She was very proud of having worked out that solution to her perpetual dilemma by herself. She had even read some of it while she had enjoyed the bar of chocolate she had picked up at the same time. Treats are good for the soul she declared as she placed it on the counter. The Saturday girl barely looked up and just put her hand out for the money. Joan didn't care she was going to enjoy the day anyway. Katie and the children would be there soon.

"Aw Mum do I have to wear a proper shirt! Can't I just wear my footie kit!"

"This dress is too small Mum sorry!"

"I don't want my hair brushed! Ow!"

One by one the children were not co-operating. Jack was still reading his Saturday paper with the tie she had picked out for him draped over the back of his chair. The appointment was at 10.30 as Matt had the inevitable match to get to in the afternoon. No one else seemed to think this portrait idea a good one. But Katie had paid her deposit and was determined her family would get there scrubbed and smart ready for a perfect family photo to adorn her walls.

"Jack, I need your help. Please!" Jack carefully folded down his paper and looked up.

"You seem to have it all under control."

"Hardly! Molly's dress doesn't fit, Lucy won't stand still for me to brush her hair and Matt won't wear anything other than a football shirt!"

"So let him."

"What?"

"Look at the brochure Katie. It says, "We capture your family just as it is. Come as you are and we will record your family magic on film for you to treasure. Wear your favourite clothes and bring accessories to express your personalities." Our family is not of the carefully brushed and washed sort. Let the children dress how they want and you will get a much better result."

Katie stared at Jack. How could he be so astute when she had missed all that? Shaking her head in wonder she turned back to her belligerent children.

"OK change of plan! You are all to dress in what you like best. Matt you can wear football kit but please make sure it is clean. Molly give me that dress for the charity bag and find something you like. And Lucy, you too can dress how you like and maybe I will pop your hair in a ponytail, OK? Oh and you all need to bring something that helps show what you like best."

The children stood, confused, looking at the strange person who had replaced their mother.

"Go on! Change! We don't have long!"

A few minutes later they were all assembled. Matt was in his clean white England kit, clutching his treasured ball that Jack had somehow managed to have signed by some of the team. Molly was wearing her new leggings and glittery top she had worn to the school disco and was holding an assortment of paintbrushes. Lucy was dressed as a witch complete with wand, cuddly black cat and broom stick. Jack was in an open necked shirt and carrying his paper; to read in the "intervals" as he put it. Katie looked down at her own "Sunday best" dress.

"Just a minute!" She raced upstairs and switched to her favourite black trousers and green shirt. She resisted the temptation to take along a rolling pin and tea towel.

Moments later as they were all piling into the car her mobile phone rang. It was Joan.

"What time are you coming dear?"

"What for Mum?"

"To pick me up?" Katie shook her head; why did her mum do this? She had made no plans to visit her today, although she would probably have popped in after the photo shoot and Matt's football game.

"Um…we are going for a family portrait Mum…I have a session booked at a studio."

"Oh how lovely! What shall I wear?"

Katie looked at her watch. They were strangely on time. She had told her family, including Jack, that they had to be at the studio at 10.00 in the hope they would make it by 10.30. As luck would have it the studio was near her mother's house.

"Whatever you are comfortable in Mum. You can watch all the photos being taken."

Katie chose to ignore Jack's sigh as she slipped into the passenger seat.

"Just a little detour. We are picking up Grandma on the way."

The photographer was obviously gifted. She had managed to make the whole experience fun for everyone. Even Jack had relaxed and joined in, striking a back-to-back pose with Matt and then swinging Lucy in the air for pictures Katie knew she would treasure. She also knew discount or no discount she was going to be spending far more than she had planned.

Their time was almost up when Joan, who had been sitting quietly on a chair in her tweed skirt and blue twinset, a relic from many years ago, spoke out.

"When is it my turn dear?" The photographer turned to Katie confused.

"You only booked a family session?"

"Well, I am family!" said Joan brightly.

"It will take time to add another adult in. I'll need to charge you for an extra fifteen minutes."

Katie looked at her mother's eager smiling face. Then at Jack's stony one. Matt was looking anxiously at the clock. Lucy made the decision for her.

"C'mon Grandma, have a go on my broomstick!"

Chapter 7

Nativity

December 2018

"Oh little town of Bethlehem how still we see thee lie…"

The little voices rang out beautifully. They might not understand all the words, but they had learnt them and were singing them clearly and loudly. Katie looked at the audience of beaming parents and sighed with relief. Not possessing much musical talent herself, she was horrified to discover her school's version of a Christmas concert was that every class rehearsed one carol and they all gathered to sing them to their parents on the last full day of term. The deputy head had explained it to her. There was to be no nativity play as that caused division and discord apparently as everyone wanted to be Mary or Joseph and no one wanted to be a sheep. And with all the teachers rehearsing their own class there was no extra burden on anyone at such a busy time. Katie thought that was a clever trick from the deputy who was nominally the music specialist in the school. At least she visited each class once before the event to play the piano for them. It was over now though. Katie had completed her first term back at work and could relax a little. The school term finished on Tuesday so she wouldn't be there for that. Instead, she would be watching the traditional nativity at Lucy's school. Lucy was playing an Angel and was very excited about her shiny wings! All she had left to do was make sure her contributions to the wall displays had been taken down and her desk drawer was tidy. Her job share would have to deal with the messy last morning, sending the children home with all their bits of paper and crushed cardboard crafts.

"Katie, can I have a word?"

It was the deputy.

"Mrs Morgan is poorly and has rung in to say she can't do tomorrow. I'm assuming you are OK to cover. It's only a half day but we can pay you a full day's supply rate. There's a nice staff get together after – the Head brings in nibbles and…"

"I'm sorry I can't."

"Are you sure?"

"Absolutely."

"Oh dear it is so hard to find supply on the last day. I would have thought you would have wanted to finish on a positive note."

"I thought I just had! I'm sorry I simply can't do tomorrow."

The deputy softened slightly. "Of course, your contribution to the carols was lovely. I must mention it to Mrs Morgan, I'm sure she would have been here today to support the class if she hadn't been ill."

Katie felt the shine slip off her triumph.

"Mummy are you coming! I have to be there on time I'm an Angel!"

"I'm ready sweetheart. I have your costume here." Katie was clutching the white dress and tin foil halo. Lucy was already wearing the wings over her uniform. As Joan was coming too, Katie had collected her while a reluctant Jack had supervised breakfast. He was going to work as normal as he had important clients to meet. He had never attended school events. He viewed that as part of Katie's "job". Katie was beginning to wonder what he saw as his role in their children's lives, but it was a conversation she was not yet ready to have. She waved as Matt left for his bus and he turned around and gave Lucy an enormous grin, "Knock 'em dead squirt!"

Lucy furrowed her brow. She did not like being called squirt. At least Matt had sort of wished her luck. She was excited. She had a whole line to say by herself. As one of the six angels that greeted the shepherds, she got to sing a whole song, just the six of them. She had practiced over and over and was sure she knew all the words. Her tummy was a jumble of nerves in a nice kind of way. She thought she would enjoy being on the stage.

Katie and Joan took their seats in the fifth row. Joan had just asked Katie for the third time what they were going to see. Katie took a breath and explained patiently.

"It's Lucy's nativity Mum. She's an Angel."

"Oh how lovely!"

The lights went down and Katie and Joan settled in their seats to watch. The child playing Joseph was struggling to remember his lines and was prompted by the donkey. There were a few nervous giggles among the parents. Maybe her deputy was right and nativities are too stressful, thought Katie as little Joseph's lip quivered. Then Mary piped up beautifully and the choir of extras at the back stood to sing the first carol as Mary, Joseph and the donkey travelled back and forth across the stage. Katie relaxed and waited for Lucy's big moment.

Lucy needed the loo. She had asked but her teacher had said there was no time. She needed to hold on until after her scene. She thought she could although the funny feeling in her tummy made her want to wee even more. The other angels were all ready. They had to hold hands as they walked on. Lucy straightened her halo that kept slipping slightly and grabbed the next angel's hand. The lights were so bright she blinked anxiously. She looked round to try to see her mummy. There she was with Grandma. She wanted to wave but remembered the teacher had been very stern when she had told them not to wave to their parents. She didn't want to get told off. Then suddenly it was her turn to speak! She took a deep breath and in her loudest voice said,

"A new King has been born and you must go to see Him!"

The song was much easier. She was easily the loudest in the group and her little voice rang clear around the hall. Her mummy and grandma were beaming and she felt happy fit to burst. They ran off to thunderous applause.

Chapter 8

Christmas

December 2018

Joan knew there was something special happening, although she couldn't quite think what. Katie had left her a note. It said 'be dressed and ready by 10.00. Molly will walk Trixie so don't worry. Please eat breakfast and give some to Trixie.' Joan thought that was odd. Katie usually told her off when she shared her breakfast with Trixie. Still, she dutifully tipped some of her cornflakes into the little dog's bowl. Trixie ignored it and barked to go outside. Joan opened the door. It was a bright crisp morning, lovely for a walk. Although it was a bit dark still. As she was up so early, she would take Trixie now.

Lucy had woken at 5.00am after a restless night hoping to spot Santa. She knew she should just go to sleep like her mummy said, 'or he wouldn't come,' it was just she so wanted to see him. She also knew she mustn't get out of bed until the rabbit ears on her clock popped up. Nor should she open her presents. She could see they were there! She had missed Santa of course but she could feel the different shapes in her stocking. She stared at the clock willing the ears to pop. It was still so dark outside. Somehow, she drifted back to sleep.

Katie was awake too. She had heard Lucy moving around and waited to see if she would settle. No sound from the other two. She didn't mind when they all got up at the crack of dawn on Christmas morning usually, but this year she was more tired than normal. She had finished wrapping and sneaking presents into the children's rooms around midnight. Matt had been the last to settle to sleep and before that she had been prepping the lunch. Jack always worked a full day on Christmas eve and had been grumpy and tired when he got home. He liked to watch a movie with her once the children had gone up and share some mince pies. He called it 'their quiet bit of Christmas'. However, it meant she was still peeling spuds at 11.00pm. She had always made their own pies, pudding and cake. This year the cake had been hastily iced at 4.00pm that day with Lucy allowed to put the decorations on. All the children had stirred the pudding and made a wish in the morning and it had steamed happily on the hob all day. In previous years those things had been done well before Christmas eve. This year between work and her mum it had all got pushed back. She had dashed over to Joan's mid-afternoon with a note of instructions for her. She did hope her mum would remember to read it. She was so tired. She slipped back to sleep.

"Mummy! Daddy! Santa's been and my rabbit ears have popped! Can we open my presents now!"

Lucy was bouncing on the bed full of excitement. Jack was yawning and Katie felt a dead weight of exhaustion pulling at her brain. She dragged herself into consciousness and smiled at Lucy.

"Go get your brother and sister then. Tell them to bring their stockings in here!"

"They are getting too big for this lark," muttered Jack. "Matt's twelve now."

"Yes, but Lucy is only five, so we have to give her the same fun we did him at this age."

"When will it stop? If we go on till she's twelve he will be nineteen and dragging a stocking from Santa into our room."

"Oh shut up Jack, let's enjoy it while it lasts!"

It was fun. The children all sat on the big king-sized bed and ripped off wrapping paper with glee. While their big presents were under the tree waiting for later after lunch, their stockings were bursting with goodies. From bright colouring pens to Barbies for Lucy, books and the sequin art for Molly, football annual and Harry Potter puzzle for Matt and much more in between. Each of them seemed happy with their haul and even Jack managed to smile at their enthusiasm. Once they had all taken their things to their rooms and Katie had gathered up the wrapping paper, she felt a strange light headedness.

"Jack, can you take all this down to the recycling bin. I just need a minute." She sat down on the bed and felt the world swim a little. "Pull yourself together Katie" she muttered and tried to force herself up. Then the world spun again and she felt sick. Not today oh please not today she thought.

Joan had been for her walk. It had been exceptionally quiet. No one was going to work it seemed. She hadn't even seen the postman on his rounds. She was tired now. She couldn't remember why she was up so early. She thought she would go upstairs for a nap. She might as well get undressed, so she didn't rumple her clothes.

Katie had forced herself to get dressed and swallow some breakfast. The children were happy with their new things and she had to get on with her day. She needed to work with military precision now. Every step in preparing lunch was timed to perfection. And she had to factor in picking up her mum and going to the morning service. They weren't normally Church goers, but Jack had been raised by staunch Church of England parents and she thought the break from excess and few moments of thinking about the true meaning of Christmas was important. Her plan was to collect her mum at 10.00. Molly would go with her and walk poor Trixie who would be left at home alone all day and they would get back in time to all walk the ten minutes to Church together. Jack might have to wrangle Lucy into some clothes though and limit how many new toys she could take with her. One Barbie was Katie's plan, although she could see Jack letting her bring two and her new cuddly horse. That might just mean extra careful watching at Church to be sure nothing was left behind.

"Come on Molly. We need to go now to get Grandma!" The turkey was already in. The oven set. Everything else lined up. If only she could shake this sick feeling.

"Jack don't let them fill up on too many sweets!" Jack grinned a chocolatey grin as he and Matt tucked into the Quality Streets.

"It's Christmas Katie! Relax!"

"Just make sure you have Lucy ready when I get back- and only one doll!"

"Where are you going?"

"To get Mum. You know I have to pick her up before Church as afterwards I will be too busy cooking."

"I could've gone to get her after."

Why oh why did Jack come out with suggestions like that when it was too late?

"She's expecting me now, so I have to go. She'll enjoy Church anyway."

"A bit of family time without your mother might've been good," muttered Jack. Katie sighed with exasperation and left, Molly trailing in her wake.

"Mum! Mum! Where are you?"

The lights were all off. Trixie was curled up in her bed and there was no sign of Joan. The breakfast dishes were still on the table though and Trixie's bowl was full of congealing cornflakes and milk.

"Throw that away Molly and find some dog food for her. When she's eaten her lead is on the hook. You will have time to get to the copse and back though do be careful. Grandma must be upstairs." Grimly Katie set off to wake her mother. She had left a note. Why couldn't Joan cooperate today of all days?

"Hello? Katie is that you?" Joan's querulous voice crossed the landing.

"Yes Mum it's me. Happy Christmas."

"Is it Christmas? How lovely! That's why no one was about!"

"What?"

"When I took Trixie out before. It was very quiet."

"Molly you don't need to…" the door slammed shut. Molly had already left.

"Come on Mum let's get you up and dressed.

"Oh come all ye faithful! Joyful and triumphant!" Katie felt a little bit triumphant after all. She had managed somehow to get Joan and Molly back in time for what had had to be a rather brisk walk to the Church. It had helped that Molly hadn't gone far saying Trixie kept sitting down and looking back towards home. It also helped that Joan's clothes were already out on her chair and she was wearing her underwear. She obviously had been up once already. She looked at Jack. He was smiling at Matt as they bellowed the loudest line of the chorus together. They looked like two cheeky little boys trying to outdo each other. Lucy was playing quietly with her Barbies; two of them but no horse. Molly was holding the hymn book with her grandma and pointing to the line they were on. Joan seemed to appreciate that and was singing happily. Katie sighed. Happy Christmas she thought Happy Christmas.

Chapter 9

Aftermath

December 2018

By Boxing Day Katie knew she was ill. Her head throbbed, her eyes stung and her throat felt like it was full of needles. Boxing Day they traditionally spent with Jack's parents. Katie knew she was never going to manage the journey to Northampton let alone a full day of her mother in law's well meant, but exhausting at the best of times, good intentions and rich food. She pleaded illness to Jack, then encouraged him that he and the children shouldn't miss out. He had looked panicked at the thought of managing all three of his children alone, until Katie pointed out they would only be in the car and then his mother would take over. She had loaded a suitable movie on the iPad for the children to watch on the way and saw them thankfully out of the door. Her last thought as she slipped back into bed was that she should have rung her mother. Instead, she switched off her phone, closed her eyes and slept.

Joan was busy. She had had a wonderful Christmas Day with Katie and she knew she would not be seeing her family on Boxing Day. Instead, her friend Katy was coming. She had been horrified to learn Katy had spent Christmas all alone and had invited her over for tea. She hummed as she shuffled around her home. She would go to the shop and get some nice cakes and things. Katie had left her a piece of Christmas cake and some mince pies, but she knew Katy loved French fancies. They often shared them on her Friday afternoon teas. She might make a few sandwiches too. Nice thin ones with the ham and turkey Katie had left her. She got it all ready and laid it out on the table. It was midday. She carefully covered the food with cling film and sat down to wait for her friend.

Katie slept all day. By the evening when the children arrived back with yet more presents and way too much sugar inside them, she managed a brief hello and goodnight before attempting a shower. She felt dizzy under the water and was soon back in bed. Jack was alarmed. It wasn't like Katie to be so ill. His mother had sent her some thick turkey soup. Katie couldn't face a single mouthful.

"Should I call a doctor?"

"It's just the flu. I need to rest. I'll be fine in a day or two."

"But what about the children?"

"You are off till New Year. I'm sure between you and the TV they will be fine. Just feed them regularly and make sure they brush their teeth once in a while." She smiled weakly at Jack's look of panic.

"What will we eat?"

"Leftovers! There's tons of food in the house. Cold turkey and ham and salad and endless cake and chocolates. You won't starve. A few vegetables might help keep them healthy and under control. Now go sleep in the spare room, you don't want to catch this."

Again, she thought of her mother as she drifted back to sleep.

Joan had a wonderful time with Katy. They had watched the Vienna concert and shared all her treats with lovely hot cups of tea Katy had made. Katy had bought her some flowers and arranged them in a vase. She had also brought a big whiteboard that she put up in Joan's living room. She said Joan could write things she needed to remember on it with the special pen. Joan had written. "Katie is ill". Jack had phoned and told her. Katy had also made little laminated cards to stick all over the kitchen. One for how to make a cup of tea, one for the toaster and one for the microwave. Then she had labelled all her cupboards with bright stickers to tell her what was inside. She had suggested she do the bedroom too, but Joan hadn't wanted to take her up there.

She felt vaguely worried it was too messy for her friend to see. She was thrilled with the kitchen. How wonderful Katy was!

Katy had loved helping the old lady. She could have gone to her cousins for Christmas but had opted instead to keep her misery to herself. A day with dear Joan was exactly what she needed; helping her made Katy feel useful again. She knew she ought to go visit the remnants of her family. They were being kind to include her. Yet if Joan's daughter was ill, she would have no one to care for her. She made her excuses to her family in her head, telling herself she would ring them later, then promised Joan she would be back in the morning. She was going to persuade her to let her help reorganise her bedroom. It was clear the old lady didn't wash her clothes often enough. She probably didn't remember what she had worn the day before. Her last label had been on the dog food. How much and how often in big letters. Poor Trixie looked thin. They had taken her for a walk in the winter sunshine and she had wolfed down the food Katy had given her. She was a very fluffy dog but under the fur there seemed very little flesh.

After three days in bed Katie needed to know how Joan was. She had dispatched Jack while the children were engrossed in "Home Alone 3". He had come back with odd tales of a tidy house, flowers, white boards and lots of labels. Apparently, Joan had told him Katie had made them. Well of course she hadn't although she wasn't going to argue. It seemed her mum could cope better than she thought.

By New Year's Day she was just about able to prepare a meal. She asked Jack to collect her mother to join them. Her favourite photo from the shoot had been delivered. She had had it framed and it sat on the floor, still wrapped and ready for a formal unveiling.

Joan was excited to see everyone and the simple fish dinner made a welcome change for everyone from the leftovers and junk fare Jack had been serving. Katie didn't eat much, although she enjoyed being up with her family. Thankfully none of them had caught her flu. She suspected she had been susceptible because she was over tired and run down. However, the rest had done her good. After dinner she asked everyone to sit on the sofa.

"I know you have all seen the album of photos from our shoot. I chose one I thought was extra special to frame and hang in the house. I want you all to see it at the same time." The children shuffled, disinterested, Joan smiled brightly. Katie pulled off the wrapping and displayed her choice. The picture had Joan seated with Jack and Katie standing behind. All three children were sitting on the floor at Joan's feet.

"Beautiful!" beamed Joan.

"Bloody typical," muttered Jack, so only Katie could hear, "look who's at the centre of the universe!"

Chapter 10

The Movies

January 2019

It was only a few days before the children returned to school and Katie felt that all she was doing was feeding the washing machine. Normally she had a rigid rota of what was to be washed on each day so she could keep on top of things. Matt sometimes disrupted it with extra football kit or Jack needed a particular shirt, but mostly it worked. Although the ironing often got left a few days. However, while she had been ill nothing had been done and she was struggling to catch up. No cleaning had been done either and again she was desperate to get the house in order before she went back to work. At the same time, she wanted to spend time with the children. Then there was her mother. She still hadn't made it to Joan's house, although they had spoken in the last few days. Joan had been bright and cheerful although her tales of "what Katy did" were increasingly baffling. Most of all she was still tired and longed to rest a little more before the term began. She kept pushing thoughts of school prep from her mind. At least the children went back a day before she did as they started on a Tuesday so she would have some space to prepare for work. Or clean the house, or finish the ironing, or visit her mother....

Matt's voice cut through her thoughts.

"Mum can we go see that movie you promised to take us to?"

"Please!" added Molly.

"Oh yes Mummy, can we, can we, please! Lucy bounced up and down with excitement.

It was rare a movie came out that all three of her children would enjoy and she had promised. She looked around at the mess, the piles of unwashed clothes, towels and bedding and sighed.

"OK let me just get a load into the machine and then we will go. Matt can you check the times for me. We may need to book."

Matt ran off gleefully to the computer and Katie scooped up Lucy's bedding. If she got that on now, then transferred it to the dryer when she got back it should be done for bedtime. She threw a few towels in to fill the load and put the rest on the floor in the utility room. It would have to wait a little longer. Just as she pressed start on the machine her phone rang.

"Hello Katie dear."

"Hello Mum."

"Um are you coming over today? I haven't seen you for ages."

"It's only been three days Mum. Remember? You came here to see the new photo of us all."

"Oh yes. I liked that picture. Still, that was three days ago. What are you doing today?"

"Mum it's on at 3.00 in 3D can we go to that one?"

Katie sighed. That would mean Lucy's bedding would never be dry for bedtime. She would have to dig out some old stuff. But it would give her time to put Matt and Molly's back on their beds if the dryer finished in time. And maybe a bit of tidying in the kitchen.

"Are you still there Katie?"

"Can we Mum?"

"Um yes I'm still here."

"Can we? I need to book as it is pretty full already."

"Yes book four tickets."

"Where are we going Katie and how do I book tickets?"

"Oh sorry Mum I was talking to Matt, I'm taking the children to the movies."

"How lovely. Can you manage on your own?"

"Of course I can, I..." Katie hesitated, recognising the soft pleading note in Joan's voice, "but some help would be lovely, do you want to come too?"

"Oh yes please!"

"Matt make that five tickets we are taking Grandma!"

Katie hung up and with a last despairing look at the washing went to put her credit card details into the booking.

The cinema foyer was crowded with hyped-up, sugar-filled youngsters pleading with exhausted parents for yet more sugar to fuel their watching. Parents with despairing eyes agreed to huge tubs of popcorn, exotic ice creams or additive laden sweets while hoping to avoid the teeth destroying drinks that would mean trips to the toilet mid film, while smug child free couples muttered their disapproval. Others queued frantically for last minute tickets or for the essential 3D glasses. Joan stood in the midst of it all looking anxiously around her.

Katie ushered her three children firmly to the ice cream stand. Joan followed obediently behind.

"One scoop each and one topping. No more no less."

"Can I have one too?"

"Of course you can Mum- what flavour would you like?"

Joan stared at the labels. She tried to focus on the words but none of them made any sense. She spotted a tub that looked as though the contents were white.

"I think I'd like that one."

Katie frowned. Since when did her mum like "Marshmallow Surprise"? Nevertheless, she ordered it with all the others and then went to get two pairs of 3D glasses. The children had theirs from last time in her handbag, she only needed some for herself and her mother.

"But I don't wear glasses Katie."

"I know Mum, it's 3D so you have to." Joan looked mystified as she followed the children past the ticket check. There were lots of numbered screens, theirs was at the far end, number 11. Lucy ran on ahead, eager not to miss anything. For a moment Katie lost sight of her as she couldn't run to catch up, because she didn't dare let go of her mother's arm and Joan was shuffling so slowly.

"Matt, go grab your sister!"

Matt disappeared in the crowd too.

"I think I need the toilet dear," said Joan as they passed the ladies. Katie frowned. She needed to locate Lucy and Matt.

"I'll stay with Grandma Mum," piped up Molly.

"Oh thanks sweetheart. Here, you hold Grandma's ice cream for her. I just need to settle Lucy and Matt in their seats and I will come back."

Joan disappeared into the toilets. There was a long queue. Katie rushed off to find Lucy and Matt. They had gone into the darkness. She looked around frantically, but Matt had remembered their seats and she saw them sitting quietly watching the adverts and eating their ice creams. She squeezed along the row to check they were Ok.

"No sweat Mum we're fine. You go get Molly and Grandma."

She smiled at Matt, squeezed apologetically back down the row and went to find Molly. She was still waiting, holding the two ice creams that were beginning to drip. She put her head round the door of the ladies. Joan was still in the queue.

"C'mon Molly let's get you seated. I'll come back for Grandma."

Molly looked doubtful but followed her mum, who watched as she slipped along the aisle to her seat and settled with the others.

She rushed back to the toilets still clutching her own and Joan's ice creams. Joan was no longer in the queue. She assumed she must be in a stall and waited patiently. Time ticked by; ice cream started to drip down her arm. There was nowhere to put Joan's down so she could use the spoon to eat her own. Instead, she held up the tub and licked round the edges. She did the same to Joan's not wanting it to run onto her clothes. She counted the people coming out. When it reached six, she started to panic. There were only six stalls. Where was her mother?

She went into the toilets and called out.

"Mum! Mum! Are you there?"

No answer. She pushed gently on each of the doors. All swung open. She ran back out into the foyer and looked around frantically. It had magically emptied as the popular films were about to start. A few teenagers hung around the concession stands planning a cool last-minute entry but there were no elderly ladies.

She wondered if Joan had somehow made her way into the screening room. She rushed back into the gloom. Casting her eyes around the packed seats there was no sign of her mother.

Two seats were empty. Either side of her children. She desperately wanted to put down the half-melted ice creams by her seat and tell her children what had happened, yet she couldn't bear the thought of pushing her way along the row another two times. Besides her mother could be anywhere by now!

She went back into the long corridor. Twelve screens, perhaps her mother had wandered into the wrong one? Sighing she decided to do this methodically and start at the top. She pushed open screen one. Some violent X rated movie was in full flow. Only a handful of men with huge tubs of popcorn were watching. She extracted herself quickly and crossed to number 2. Cleaners were working their way down the aisles. No Joan. Number 3 was the same. But number four was packed with young children and mothers engrossed in the latest Disney Princess offering. She cast her eyes around the gloom. It was impossible to make out faces. She climbed the stairs looking along the rows. No Joan.

By the time she reached screen 8 she had ditched the ice creams and was contemplating asking the management for help. Her movie would be starting any second and her children were alone. She realised she had their 3D glasses too. Frustrated and panicked she pushed open the door. Sitting alone in the front row intent on the advert for men's deodorant was Joan. Taking a deep breath to try to calm her temper she rushed over.

"Katie I was wondering where you all were?" Joan beamed. Katie felt all the anger slip away at her mum's happy, smiling face.

"There's been a slight change of plan Mum. We are in a different room. The children are already there. C'mon let's go." She helped her mum up. They walked into number 11 just as the opening credits started to a blare of loud orchestral sound. Joan started at the noise. Katie hurried her along to their seats while neighbouring customers muttered under their breath. She asked the children to shuffle up, so she was next to Joan. No way was she letting her out of her sight again. She pulled glasses out of her bag and passed them down to the children before offering a set to her mother.

"But I don't wear glasses."

Dragons and serpents swooped and circled towards Joan. Huge birds glided above her. The booming, clanging music startled her and she shrank away frightened. She took off the glasses and it all faded into a fuzzy mess. Much better.

"Put your glasses back on Mum." hissed Katie.

"But I don't…" said Joan, loudly so Katie could hear.

"Shh," said an angry voice behind her, making her jump.

"Just wear your glasses and enjoy the movie Mum."

Joan sighed and put the awful glasses back on. A lion roared right in her face. She started and closed her eyes. That was better. That made it all go away. Katie was engrossed in the screen and didn't notice. Joan thought she would just keep her eyes closed until it was all over.

Katie saw her mother's closed eyes. She sighed; Her mum had obviously dozed off. What a waste of a ticket. Still, it wasn't really her cup of tea either. Perhaps she should follow suit. After all she was still so very tired from being ill. Despite the noise she drifted off.

Matt was laughing. "Mum! Grandma! wake up! The movie is over."

Molly was worried. "Are you OK Mum?"

Katie shook herself awake, "Yes I'm fine sweetheart. I don't know how I slept through all that noise. Is Lucy Ok?"

"I need the toilet Mummy!"

"I'll take her," said Joan. "I wasn't asleep just resting my eyes."

"Um no Mum I will take her thanks, I need to go too. Could you go with Molly and Matt into the foyer?" Katie looked pointedly at Matt hoping he would understand he needed to hang on to his grandma. Matt hadn't got it at all and was heading swiftly towards the exit.

"Mummy come on I need a wee!"

"Don't worry Mum I'll hold Grandma's hand so neither of us get lost." Katie smiled gratefully at her older daughter and took Lucy's hand as they moved quickly to the exit. The toilet queue was massive and Katie grew more and more anxious as they waited their turn. Lucy hopped from foot to foot. They squeezed into a stall together in the end, although by then Katie was far too worried about Joan to go herself and fairly dragged Lucy out into the foyer as soon as her hands were washed.

"Mummy I haven't dried my hands!"

"Never mind sweetheart the queue for the dryers was too long."

"But you always make me use them even though I hate the noise."

"Today's your lucky day then don't complain."

Lucy started at the sharp tone in Katie's voice. What had she done to make Mummy cross?

"There they are!" Katie almost wept with relief as she practically dragged Lucy to where the others were waiting.

"C'mon squirt you took forever!" Matt grumbled.

Lucy's face crumpled, why was Matt was being mean as well. It didn't look like Mummy would even tell him off. She had her "I'm too busy to deal with you face," on and was guiding Grandma towards the exit while still holding Lucy's hand much too tightly. This hadn't been so much fun as she had thought it would be. Some bits of the movie had been too scary. She didn't like the lion when it fought the dragon as its claws had been too close to her face. Even though she knew it was only a movie, it had all seemed very big and real and she would have liked to have sat next to Mummy and held her hand in the scary bits. Yet Mummy had sat with Grandma and she had been stuck with Matt who just laughed at the danger. Now Mummy was inexplicably cross with her and Matt was calling her squirt. Sometimes nothing made sense anymore.

Chapter 11

GP Appointment

January 2019

The night after the trip to the movies, Katie lay awake for hours pondering her mother's state of health. Obviously, her mother had memory issues, but what she found hardest was the way Joan would cover up her mistakes. Surely, she must have known she was in the wrong screen. Over and over again there would be that bright smile and positive voice saying she was OK. And yet she wasn't OK. And what about all those stickers and signs all over her house. Her mother had managed to organise herself so carefully. Yet instead of admitting it she told Jack that she, Katie, had done it. That made no sense at all. Her mother had always been a healthy eater and now she was stuffing herself with chocolate and ice cream. That was more than just not remembering how to cook. It didn't add up at all. Unable to sleep Katie crept downstairs and did what she knew she should have done long ago. She clicked on the computer screen and googled "Dementia."

Jack found Katie slumped in the study chair with the computer clicking and whirring on the Alzheimer's society pages. Gently he nudged her awake.

"How long have you been there?"

"I couldn't sleep. Mum was so odd today. I, I decided to do some research."

"About time," muttered Jack.

"It's not easy…she is all I have!"

"No, she isn't! You have me and the kids. It's more like you are all she has and you feel responsible. Then with all your other responsibilities you don't have time to deal with it, so you bury your head in the sand and hope it will go away."

"Oh Jack don't be so mean."

Jack ran his hands through his hair and furrowed his brow. Katie used to find that gesture endearing as it usually meant he was trying hard to find the right way to say something without upsetting her. She waited.

"I'm not, I'm being honest and it is time someone was. I'm glad you have started to accept what is happening. Now we need to get some help, so you don't have to manage alone."

"What do you suggest. I've read so much tonight and there is no obvious path to take. I don't even know what kind of dementia she has."

"Well maybe that is where we start."

"How?"

"Where do you go to start with any kind of medical problem?"

"The GP?"

"Yes! So, let's make an appointment."

"But how do I do that? It isn't for me after all it's for Mum."

"Do you know who her GP is?"

"Yes."

"Then phone and make an appointment. The receptionist won't know you aren't her and you know all your mum's details after all."

Katie nodded. That was the easy part. She looked Jack straight in the eye.

What if she won't come."

"Then you have to persuade her sweetheart. That I'm afraid is up to you."

In the end Katie had been honest with the receptionist, telling her she was concerned about her mother's failing memory and odd behaviour. Booking an appointment hadn't been an issue and Katie had been advised to come along. The receptionist had booked her with the GP best known for dealing with dementia patients and had warned he could only do an initial test. If he then felt it necessary, he would refer her on to the memory clinic. Satisfied she had finally put things in motion Katie put a big red ring around the date on her calendar. She had two weeks to convince her mother to go to see her GP.

She left it until two days before the appointment. Getting the children back to school and herself back into work consumed her life and while she spoke to or visited her mother every day, she didn't have time to sit down and broach what she knew would be a sensitive subject. Nevertheless, when the date loomed large, she knew she had to speak to Joan. She decided to go over first thing in the morning on a bright sunny day and suggest they take Trixie for a walk. Her mother had always loved to walk and talk. Somehow it seemed easier to Katie, to have something physical to do while telling her mother she was losing her mind.

Joan however had not got out of bed when Katie let herself in. She fed Trixie and let her out in the garden, carefully ticking the box on the chart for feeding the dog. It had plenty of gaps and Trixie still looked thin. Then she tidied the kitchen and mopped the floor, hoping her mother would wake naturally. By 10.00 it was obvious she wasn't going to and Katie did not want to spend the whole day on her mother's chores. She went slowly upstairs and knocked tentatively on her mother's door.

"Who is it? Who's there? I have a dog you know!"

"It's OK Mum it's only me," Katie pushed open the door and smiled at her mother. Joan somehow looked smaller, shrunken even in the big, crumpled bed.

"Katie! What are you doing here in the dead of night?"

"Oh Mum, it isn't nighttime at all; it's half way through the morning!"

Joan looked set to argue so Katie pulled back the curtains to let the winter sun stream in.

"See Mum It's a lovely day. Why don't I run you a nice bath and when you are dressed, we can go for a long walk with Trixie."

Joan looked to protest but Katie was already halfway out the door.

"I'll bring you a cup of tea first Mum OK," she called over her shoulder.

Joan seemed to take forever to dress. Katie had carefully pulled clean clothes out of the wardrobe, popping any she thought dirty into a bag to load the machine while her mum washed. As usual there was nothing in the laundry basket. When Joan appeared, her unfamiliar jumper was on back to front.

"Oh Mum, let me help you."

"Why what's wrong?" said Joan defensively.

"I must have put your jumper out upside down. You have it on back to front."

"Do I? Oh dear. I don't remember this one. Is it mine?"

"Yes Mum, I gave it to you for Christmas."

"Oh how lovely, thank you dear."

Last year's Christmas that is, thought Katie, not this year. This year I gave you a blouse. Suddenly unable to postpone another minute Katie seized the opportunity.

"Mum, I need to ask you to do something for me?"

"Of course dear, what do you need?"

"Well, we have all noticed how you have been forgetting things a lot lately. And getting lost a bit. Like when we went to the cinema and you went into the wrong screen." Joan looked at her blankly clearly unable to recall that particular experience.

"Well, it must be horrible for you, not being able to remember things properly."

"Oh it is Katie, it is! I don't know what's happening to me. I don't know where I am or who I am half the time. I can't even remember what day it is. What's happening to me?"

Shocked by her mother's unexpected, distressed candour Katie was wrong footed into saying too much.

"I think you might have dementia Mum."

The words hung in the air between them. Joan's face quivered and then closed.

"Don't be so silly Katie. I am not losing my marbles like some decrepit old lady. I'm just a bit forgetful that's all!"

Kicking herself for going too far, Katie tried desperately to back pedal, "No one is saying you are old and decrepit Mum. Far from it. You are just a bit forgetful and we need to find out why. I…I spoke to the doctor's surgery. They would like to see you, have a chat…"

"I'm not seeing a doctor! He will want to put me away! Is that what you want? Put me in a home so you can have all my money! How dare you!"

Katie was about to shout back when pages from her research floated into her mind. "Remember however afraid you are the dementia sufferer is more afraid. And their anger is usually a way to cover their fear."

She forced a gentle smile and took her mother's hand.

"No one is sending you anywhere. I won't let them! I will be right there with you Mum every step of the way. Wouldn't it be lovely if we could know why you are forgetting things? Maybe even find a way to fix it?"

She sensed her mother softening.

"Could they fix it?"

Katie knew the answer to that question. Unless her mother's problem wasn't dementia, rather a physical problem like a tumour, there would be no cure. However, getting her to the doctor seemed to be worth a little white lie.

"Perhaps Mum, perhaps," she whispered.

As it turned out getting Joan to the doctors was very easy. On the day Katie simply turned up and reminded Joan it was the day of her appointment. True to form Joan acted as though she knew that all along and left happily with her daughter. Only when they had arrived at the surgery and were waiting to go in, did Joan start to raise doubts.

"So why am I here Katie? I'm not ill."

Determined not to upset Joan, Katie was evasive, "Let's just wait and see what the doctor wants shall we?"

"Oh, did she ask to see me?"

"We are seeing a male doctor Mum."

"But I always see the lady doctor. Doctor German."

"Well today you are seeing Doctor Fish."

"Why?"

"I think Doctor German could be on holiday," Katie improvised.

"Well why don't we come back when she's home. Whatever it is I'm sure it can wait."

"No Mum it can't. It has to be today."

"But I don't want to see a different doctor. I want to go home." Joan got up and headed towards the door.

"Please don't go Mum. Doctor Fish is very nice and I have come over especially to take you. Just stay for me won't you."

Joan fixed Katie with a fierce stare.

"Why do you have to come with me? I'm not a child you know."

"You...you asked me to Mum, so I made special arrangements. Do sit back down please it must be nearly our turn."

"Oh all right. But there's nothing wrong with me."

As Joan sat down at last Katie noticed all eyes in the waiting room were on them. Most registered sympathy, a few amusement and a couple turned away embarrassed by the scene. Katie tried not to react and simply reached over and held her mother's hand.

"It's Ok Mum, not long now."

"Joan Jessup to room 5 please."

"Oh that's me. Come on then Katie let's go see what Dr German wants me for!"

"It's Doctor...oh never mind."

"Hello Mrs Jessup, do take a seat."

Joan obediently sat and smiled broadly at the doctor.

"So, what seems to be the problem?"

"You tell me doctor you wanted to see me!"

"Er well no you made an appointment?"

"Only because you asked me to!"

"Ok...well...do you have any symptoms."

"No, I'm fit as a flea!"

The doctor glanced at Katie who was desperately trying to get his attention without her mother realising.

"Perhaps your friend can help?"

"I'm her daughter actually and..."

"Katie," interjected Joan," this is Katie my daughter." She beamed again.

"Well perhaps Katie can help us get to the bottom of the problem."

"Is there a problem?"

"Mum has an issue with her memory," blurted Katie, "she forgets things and gets lost sometimes."

"I see."

"It's not that bad." Joan crossed her arms defensively and glared at her daughter. "She's exaggerating."

"Well," said the doctor smiling at them both, "How about I ask you a few simple questions and we can tell how bad the problem is."

Joan glanced at Katie nervously.

"Go on Mum it will help you to know. Then we can fix things."

The doctor pursed his lips about to contradict Katie then thought better of it and instead reached for a well-worn book from his shelf.

"This is a standard memory test. Let's see how you get on. Some of the questions might seem very simple but I need you to answer them all."

"Like a test in school?" asked Joan, "I was good at those!"

"Yes, just like that Mum."

"What is your full name?"

"Joan Rosemary Jessup."

Joan happily reeled off her date of birth and full address including her postcode. She counted down in 4's from 90 and correctly identified some shapes and even copied them rather shakily, yet still legibly, at the doctor's request. Katie was beginning to wonder if she had made a mistake in bringing her when the doctor asked Joan the name of the road they were in.

"I don't know I've never been here before."

Katie stared at her mum; this had been her surgery for about 40 years. She went to speak but the doctor held up his hand and went on.

"Can you tell me the date Joan?"

"It's Wednesday!"

"Do you know what month it is?"

"I think its April, yes it's April!"

"Ok, can you tell me the year?"

"Yes, its…oh yes 1986 of course!"

Katie stared in disbelief, saying nothing.

"Now Joan one last question. I'm going to tell you the name of 3 things, then time 2 minutes and see if you can remember them. Is that OK?"

"Yes, I'm ready."

Joan furrowed her brow concentrating hard as the doctor said, "Chair, velvet, flower." He repeated it again and then moved on to the next question while his phone timed two minutes. Joan was happily identifying animal pictures when the beep sounded.

"Now Joan can you remember the three things?"

Joan looked anxiously at Katie.

"Don't help her please," he said sharply, "it is your test after all Joan," he said more gently. "I can give you a clue. One is a piece of furniture."

"Oh yes! A chair!" Joan beamed delightedly.

"Yes," said the doctor, "well done. The next is a type of material."

"Cotton?"

"Softer than cotton."

"No…I don't remember."

"OK never mind. The last one was something pretty, smells nice too."

"Perfume!"

The doctor smiled. "Just give me a minute and I will add up your score."

Joan looked worried as the doctor totted up the numbers he had made on his pad.

"Don't worry Mum it will be OK." Katie tried to reassure her mother while the knot of panic in her own stomach tightened.

"Well Joan you scored 21 out of 25 which is very good. However, a few of your answers concern me. You couldn't remember any of the words after 2 minutes without help and then only one of them. That could just be age related as we all get more forgetful with age. The biggest concern was that you had no idea what time of year it was or which year."

"Didn't I?"

"No, you said it was April when it is January. We have only just had Christmas. Do you remember that now?"

"Oh yes of course I went to Katie's house!"

"OK…and you didn't know where you were and yet you have been a patient here for a very long time according to my records. Although you and I haven't met before."

"No, I usually see Dr German. Katie made me see you today."

"Yes, yes you do. You have done an excellent job in your test with me today."

Joan basked in his praise.

"Would you do something else for me Joan? You see I think your daughter is a bit worried about your memory and I think I know a special doctor who can help you more than I can. I would like to refer you to the memory clinic. They can fully diagnose what is happening. Why you forget some things. Would you go with Katie to see her?"

Joan furrowed her brow again and looked at Katie.

"I think we should Mum. We'll go together."

"Oh alright. If you both think I should."

"I'll do the referral today, although it might take a while to come through. In the meantime, you can get some aids to help your mum. There are clocks on the market that give days and dates as well as time. And putting some simple instructions up around the house for daily tasks might be useful. I doubt your mum cooks very much now, so looking at some convenience food might be wise.

Most importantly, I would suggest she doesn't go far alone. Her orientation seems to be the most affected area so far. I'll give you some leaflets that might help with ideas for support."

Katie's brain stuck on the words "so far," how far was this going to go, she wanted to ask. Instead, she simply smiled at the doctor, took the leaflets and helped her mum to the door.

"Thank you doctor," she and Joan chorused in unison.

Joan held Katie's arm as she walked unsteadily out of the clinic.

"Am I going to be alright?" she asked, her voice quavering.

"Yes Mum, I will make sure you are alright," whispered Katie, patting her mum's arm." Don't worry, I'm here."

Chapter 12

Lucy's Spellings

February 2019

Lucy chewed the end of her pencil. The teacher was standing at the front of the class ready to begin. She had followed all her instructions; written the numbers 1-5 down the page, drawn a neat line with a ruler and put her name and the date at the top in her very best handwriting. She hoped that would be enough.

"Number 1- dog," said the teacher.

Lucy furrowed her brow, surely that was d-o-g. She wrote it down quickly. The teacher was repeated it. Yes, she was sure she had that one right. Relief flooded her body.

"Number 2- Super."

Lucy concentrated hard. Break it down to how it sounds she thought. That's what they tell us. What makes those sounds. S…must be oo…p…er! That would be it Sooper! But it didn't look quite right.

"Number 3- people."

Lucy wanted to cry. She had no idea where to start. It must be a "p" Then maybe 'ee' but she knew there were other ways of making that sound too. They had learnt that in phonics last week. It could be 'ea'. She crossed out her first attempt and tried again. 'Pea'. What came next? She started to panic. The end of the word sounded like 'pul', but 'peapul' didn't look right at all. She crossed it out again and started over. The teacher was moving on to number 4. Lucy didn't hear her; she was trying desperately to get the letters to behave and look like the right word. Realising she had missed a word she glanced over at her nearest classmate to see what they were writing.

"Lucy keep your eyes on your own work!"

Lucy put her head down on the desk and gave up.

The teacher was holding her spelling test and looking down at her kindly. Still Lucy knew she was cross. She knew that tone of voice grown-ups use when they are trying to sound nice but were actually going to use mean words. Her mummy did it sometimes. When she was disappointed with Lucy. When she hadn't tidied her room or brushed her teeth properly. She looked down at the ground and waited for the words to hit.

"First of all, Lucy do you understand why it is wrong to look at someone else's work in a test?" Lucy said nothing, knowing it was pointless to try to explain she had only missed a word and wanted to know what it was. She wasn't actually cheating at all, yet somehow she knew the teacher wouldn't understand that. When she didn't answer the teacher carried on.

"It's called cheating. And it doesn't help you. If you had copied Tracey's work, how would I know if you could spell Tuesday or not."

Tuesday, thought Lucy, so that was the word I missed. I couldn't spell it anyway, so it didn't really matter if I looked at Tracey's paper or not. She stared at her desk and said nothing.

"It seems to me," droned the teacher, "that you hadn't actually practiced your spellings at all this week, had you?"

Lucy looked up. She thought through the week. Monday Mummy had been to work and so Lucy went to after school club. That meant by the time they got home Mummy was all flustered and only had time to cook dinner and chase the children into bed. Tuesday, they had rushed over to Grandma's after school to fix her telly again. Why Grandma didn't just buy a new one Lucy didn't understand at all. Maybe Grandma was very poor? Anyway, that had meant a late tea and Mummy had gone all quiet and looked worried, so she hadn't wanted to bother her about spellings. Wednesday Mummy had decided they could go to the park after school to make up for Tuesday and by Thursday Lucy had forgotten all about the spelling test. Until now. Until the teacher had said it was time to write the numbers down the page. Lucy thought all that but said nothing. She didn't want to get into more trouble.

"You must stay in at break and practice these words. Then I shall put a note in your book bag for your mother. Perhaps next week you will do better."

Lucy sat at her desk copying out the five words over and over. Every few minutes she looked up and glanced out the window. She could see all her friends running about. It was her class's turn on the adventure playground today. They only got one break time a week on there. Now she had missed out. A tear rolled down her cheek. Spellings were stupid.

At the end of the day the teacher put a sealed envelope in Lucy's bookbag. She was going to after school club so the teacher couldn't talk to her mummy. She knew the letter would say she had been cheating. She hadn't. Not really. All through the club activities Lucy wondered what to do. She could throw the letter in the bin then Mummy would never read it and never know the teacher had been cross. She knew that was the wrong thing to do. Although on Fridays Mummy was always so tired and grumpy. She definitely didn't want her to see it today. Maybe she should just hide it till Sunday. On Sundays Mummy and Daddy had a lie in as Matt would put a DVD on for Lucy in the morning and Mummy was usually happier after that. Yes, she would leave it in her bag and give it to Mummy on Sunday.

Katie was concerned. Lucy was very quiet on the way home from school. Even the after-school care ladies had noticed and wondered if she was poorly. Lucy had said she was fine and had even put her book bag away carefully, not left it strewn in the hall like usual. Katie always tried to remember to check the children's bags for notes and homework as she knew how quickly children forgot things. Matt had a note about yet another football match, Molly had a page of maths to do for the weekend. Then there was a letter in Lucy's bag. Katie tore it open anxiously, her mother instincts telling her it wasn't going to be good.

"Lucy! Can you come here a minute please?"

Lucy crept down the stairs. She could see the letter in Mummy's hand. She didn't want to be told off again. It wasn't fair. She had already missed the adventure playground. She stood in front of her mother, eyes down and anxious.

"Lucy, sweetheart, it's OK."

Lucy looked up. Hadn't Mummy read the letter? She stared mutely at Katie.

"Your teacher tells me you had a spelling test today and we hadn't practiced. I'm so sorry sweetheart I hadn't realised you had spellings to learn. We were so rushed last weekend I didn't check your bag. I have the new ones here in this envelope. I will make sure we do them every day so next time you will get them all right."

Lucy looked suspiciously at her mother. Was that it? No telling off.

Katie wrapped her arms around her smallest child. When had life got so hard for her little girl? She was going to ring that school first thing Monday morning and give them a piece of her mind! Lucy was far too young to be expected to manage all alone. Surely the teacher knew that if homework wasn't done at her age it had to be down to the parents. She bristled with annoyance at the tone of the letter. With three children, her mother and a job, sometimes things got missed. She pushed away her rising sense of guilt and focussed on the bad teaching methods. Punishing a lively young child by keeping her in was ridiculously counterproductive. Lucy was not a cheat!

"Come on sweetheart, let's see if we can find you a glass of milk and some biscuits. Then we will have a go at these words. OK?"

Lucy stared at her mother and nodded. She wasn't quite sure how this had happened. Mummy wasn't cross after all and she was getting biscuits before dinner. She followed her mother meekly into the kitchen. Sometimes grown-ups made no sense at all.

On Monday morning Katie was at work and never made that call.

Chapter 13

The Park

February 2019

"Hello? Katie?"

"Hello Mum."

"Are you coming over today?"

"Yes Mum it's Tuesday I always come on a Tuesday."

"Oh good. Are you coming now?"

Since the visit to the doctor, Katie had developed a routine. On workdays she would ask Molly to say hello to Grandma on the way to school and remind her that Katie wouldn't be available that day. Molly would tell Grandma to write it down. Katie felt bad about putting such pressure on her child, although Molly didn't seem to mind and would chat happily to Joan all the way to school. Then on the days Katie didn't work she had some strict rules. She recognised she was going to have to help her mother manage everyday tasks. However, she needed it to not be at the expense of her family anymore. She never went to Joan's until her day's washing was done and in the dryer. That usually meant getting up a bit earlier and loading it before she took the girls. That also gave her time to do some cleaning in her own home while it washed. On Tuesdays she helped her mother with her own washing, on Wednesdays they did their shopping together and Thursdays she would help her mother clean and tidy her house. Each day she would sit down for a healthy lunch with Joan and make her a sandwich for later. She always left in plenty of time to prepare her family's meal and would send Joan off for a walk with the dog when she left. Her last act was to make sure the TV was on for Joan when she returned from her walk and the little dog had fresh food and water. It was exhausting, yet it was working. At least on those three days. She tried not to think about the other four days too much.

"No Mum a bit later."

"Oh, it's just my telly isn't working."

"I know Mum, I will sort it when I arrive."

"I think it's broken."

"Yes, I know, I am good at fixing it."

"Really?"

"Oh yes." Katie had been reading and the advice was to reassure and encourage. If her mother was fixated on the TV being broken, when in reality all she needed to do was press "Sky", even though she didn't have Sky anymore, there was no way Katie would ever change her mind. That was what the experts said so Katie was going with it.

And distract. That was another good technique.

"Why don't you read the paper?"

"I haven't got one."

"Well pop round to the shop and get one. By the time you have read it I will be there."

"Ok see you later."

Katie went back to cleaning the manky depths of Matt's bedroom. She didn't venture in very often and there had been a smell emanating from the wardrobe she needed to investigate. She had found a rotting apple core, a sticky chocolate wrapper and a half-eaten sandwich in an old backpack on top of a good pair of jeans that were absolutely smothered in mud stuffed behind the clean clothes. Clearly Matt had been somewhere he shouldn't in his new jeans and rather than face the music he had hidden the evidence. Once she had started in his room, she knew she wouldn't stop until she had it straight. She grimaced at the thought. However, it had to be done.

Joan had hung up the phone feeling vaguely disappointed. She thought Katie was coming over today. With the telly not working what was she going to do? Trixie barked. Joan looked outside. It seemed like a nice day. She went and got the dog's lead. She determined to go back to the park for once instead of just down to the copse and back.

Katie felt shattered as she shovelled her washing into the dryer. After dealing with Matt's mess all she wanted was to sit down and have a cuppa. However, she knew she needed to get to Joan's house if she was going to get her washing done and in the dryer before she had to get back. She sighed. This routine was jolly hard work! She pulled herself up, grabbed her handbag and set off.

Joan was enjoying a lovely walk. The air was crisp, Trixie was clearly having a wonderful time sniffing all the doggy smells and she relished her success in managing the outing. They had circled the park 3 times and she was considering a fourth.

"Hello? It's Joan, isn't it?"

Joan looked at the smiling lady. She had no idea who she was.

"It's Elaine. We met up here a few times walking the dogs. My Susie and your Trixie had such fun together. I haven't seen you for a while. Are you OK?"

"Yes, I'm fine. How are you?"

"Good, really good. Are you arriving or leaving?"

"Oh, I just got here!"

"Lovely. Shall we walk together?"

"How nice. Yes let's."

Joan spent the next hour walking round the park while the stranger told her all about her grandchildren. It was very pleasant even if a bit odd. When Elaine said she had to go home, Joan felt rather sad. Trixie looked exhausted and she had some vague feeling she needed to be somewhere else. Oh yes! Her TV was broken! The man was coming to repair it!

"Well, it was lovely to see you again Joan. Hopefully it won't be so long before we bump into each other again."

"Yes, that would be nice. I must be going now though as the TV man is coming."

"Bye then."

"Bye!"

Joan hurried home. She hoped she hadn't missed the repair man. What time did he say he was coming? She opened her door.

"Katie! What a wonderful surprise!"

Chapter 14

The Audition

February 2019

"I have to tell you something!" Lucy tugged at her mother's sleeve while Katie carried on staring at the emails on her phone as the girls came out of school. Nothing important, just the usual junk. She snapped her phone shut and turned to her youngest child who was now hopping from foot to foot with impatience.

"What is it Lucy?"

"I've been chosen!"

"For what?"

"To sing silly!"

"What is "silly singing"?"

"No Mummy you are silly!"

"Don't be rude Lucy."

Lucy bit her lip. This wasn't going at all right. She had been so excited and now Mummy was spoiling it. She tried again.

"I had a dition."

"Huh?" Katie's phone pinged again and she quickly checked the text. Molly was late out and they needed to get over to her mother's. Joan had been ringing all day about her television again. Katie had too much school prep to do as well as an ironing mountain and hadn't made it over there. Now Jack was checking he could invite a new client for drinks on Saturday. Then a restaurant meal. She was relieved; no cooking. She knew schmoozing clients was part of his job, although she hated it when she had to host. She thumbed a quick OK. There was Molly at last!

"C'mon girls we need to get to Grandma's."

"I don't want to go!" shouted Lucy. "We always have to go to Grandma's! I want to go home! I need to practice!"

"Practice what?"

"I told you!"

"Oh, the silly singing thing…you can do that later."

"No!"

"Lucy stop being awkward. Grandma needs our help. And there will be biscuits." Katie hated it when her children made a scene in public so a little bit of bribery might just smooth it over. Why was Lucy being so difficult?

Lucy however was beyond soothing with biscuits. She covered her face with her hands and burst into tears.

Katie stopped. She put her phone in her pocket and crouched down to Lucy's level.

"Whatever is the matter, Lucy?" she coaxed gently.

"I was picked and you spoiled it."

"I don't understand. Tell me from the beginning."

Lucy peeped out from behind her hands. Her face was all blotchy from crying and her nose was running. She sniffed and wiped her face on her sleeve. Katie resisted the urge to correct and instead reached into her pocket for a tissue. She gently wiped Lucy's eyes and then her nose.

"Blow!" Lucy obeyed. "That's better. Now tell me what has got you so upset?"

Lucy looked suspiciously at her mother. Why was she suddenly being all nice? Was it another attempt to persuade her to go to Grandma's? She liked biscuits and she liked Grandma, but this was too important.

"I went to Mrs McCarthy at lunchtime. We all had to sing on our own. She picked me."

"What for?"

"To sing of course!"

"When Lucy? When do you have to sing?"

"In the Church. Everyone else sings the chorus but I sing the verse. Just me!"

"That sounds lovely dear. When is this happening?"

Lucy looked blankly at her mother. Why was that important? Mrs McCarthy had told her to go home and practice for the 'Big Day', so that was what she was going to do.

"I think can help Mum." Molly had been watching silently as Mum had been so awful and Lucy had thrown her tantrum. She had seen the looks on the other children's faces as they walked past. And the parents. She just wanted to get out of there. Hopefully, she could fix this.

"There were auditions at lunchtime. All the children who wanted to sing in the choir went along. I didn't go as I don't really like singing. I suppose Lucy must have. They are probably starting to get ready for the Easter service in the Church. We have one every year you know."

"Easter! But that's weeks away. Loads of time to practice."

"Miss said I had to do it now!"

"OK Lucy how about you sing your song in the car on the way to Grandma's?"

"I need you to help me to learn the words!"

"Molly can sit next to you and help you can't you Molly?"

"Course I can Lucy? C'mon show me the words. I'll help you." Anything to get out of the empty playground. The caretaker was standing by the gate waiting to lock up. Molly had hoped to get her homework done before dinner so she could watch a new show everyone at school was talking about. Now she guessed she would end up missing it. She took her little sister's hand firmly and walked towards the gate.

As they sat in the car Lucy hugged her hurt feelings to herself. She didn't feel like singing now.

"What a lovely surprised!" exclaimed Joan when she opened the door. "Come in- I'll put the kettle on. I have some biscuits somewhere girls and some juice."

"I can help you Grandma," said Molly, "Mum can get on and fix your TV."

"There's nothing wrong with my TV!"

Katie bit back her frustration as Molly shot her an uncharacteristic venomous look.

"Grandma gets lonely and confused just go get your juice," she hissed at Molly.

"So, Mum how has your day been?"

"Oh fine, nothing special."

"Did you go for a walk with Trixie?" The little dog was running around and around in circles barking wildly.

"Of course I did. I always do." Joan snapped defensively. "Stop that Trixie!"

"OK Mum, I was just making conversation." Katie had never heard Joan speak so harshly to the dog. Her brow furrowed. She was pretty sure Trixie was not getting the exercise or regular meals she needed. However, Joan had always adored her and at least she was some kind of company. She pushed unwelcome thoughts from her brain and smiled at her mother.

"Lucy has been chosen to sing a solo in the Easter service Mum. Isn't that exciting!"

"How lovely. Is it soon?"

"Easter Mum, a few weeks yet." Katie swallowed, her mother was so unaware of days and dates lately. The doctor's face swum into her mind; it couldn't be much longer until their date at the memory clinic came up.

Lucy bounced into the room, "would you like to hear me sing it Grandma?"

"Of course."

Lucy took a deep breath, beamed at her audience and launched into her solo.

Joan watched delighted and when Lucy reached the chorus she joined in with gusto. Katie smiled and started to relax. What a wonderful way for Lucy to practice. Somehow her mum had saved the day.

Molly sighed, grabbed Trixie's ball and took her outside to play. She had had enough of the Lord of the Dance for one day!

Chapter 15

Easter Service

March 2020

Lucy was wildly excited if a little bit nervous. It was The Big Day! She was going to sing her solo at the Easter service. Grandma had been amazing helping her practice every week. She had never thought her grandma knew anything about music, yet she knew all the words to the song. She hadn't needed to look at the words even once. Lucy understood Grandma forgot stuff a lot but obviously not everything. Lucy remembered the words now too and was sure she would be able to sing it well. They had practiced at the Church the day before where she even got to use a microphone. Her voice sounded a bit strange and extra loud, although she got used to it by the end. Mummy had washed and ironed her uniform and even made her have a hair wash the night before. On a school night! Usually, hair only got washed at the weekend. Obviously being chosen to sing was a 'Really Big Deal', even if Mummy hadn't thought so at the start.

"Good morning Lucy, now don't you look smart! I will take you both to school a bit early and then go and get Grandma so she can see you sing too. Eat your breakfast quickly. You can go to the last bit of breakfast club like on the days I work."

"If you don't go straight to the Church, you won't get a good seat!" All the mums would drop their children and then go across the road and take their places. Latecomers were squeezed into back pews or even had to stand.

"Don't worry sweetheart, I have spoken to Mrs McCarthy about how Grandma has helped you practice and needs to see you sing. She has reserved us two seats on the front row."

Lucy frowned. She wanted Mummy to see, however the front row was a bit close. She decided not to let it bother her. She would just look at Grandma and imagine they were still in her front room practicing.

"C'mon then girls brush your teeth quick and let's go."

Joan was waiting on the doorstep. Katie had set her alarm to wake her and put a huge notice by her bed to remind her it was Lucy's Church service. Her clothes had been laid out by her bed so she could get dressed. Katie had chosen a rather old fashioned, yet still smart, blue suit from the back of her wardrobe for her. Joan hadn't worn it for ages. The zip on the skirt didn't do up for some reason but the jacket hung down over it so no one would know. She just needed to remember to hold onto her skirt when she walked so it didn't fall down. She had some pennies in her purse for the collection and a clean white handkerchief. She wasn't entirely sure what the occasion was and she thought there might have been something else she should have done. However, she did know today was 'Very Important' and she had to be ready.

"Hello Mum don't you look smart. Let's get in the car. Have you had some breakfast?"

"Of course!" Joan lied, realising that eating was what she had forgotten. Never mind she could eat later, Katie was clearly in a hurry.

At the Church they took their seats in the front row. Katie had noticed with alarm that her mother's zip wasn't fastened. She groaned inwardly realising she had chosen an outfit too small since her mother had been gaining weight. She still couldn't understand that when Joan seemed to eat so little. Nor why her mother hadn't chosen something different to wear when she realised. She couldn't worry about that now as the children were coming in.

The service was delightful with readings and songs from all the classes as well as the choir. There was even a lovely moment when the youngest children danced in the aisles. Lucy sang all the choir songs with a smile on her face. Her big moment was coming after the Vicar's talk. So far she looked relaxed and happy, not nervous at all. Joan was smiling and enjoyed singing along to the congregations' hymns. What a lovely morning Katie thought to herself.

"And now we will have our final hymn, 'The Lord of the Dance,' with a special solo by Lucy." The Headmistress smiled encouragingly, as Lucy took her place behind the microphone. She looked down at her grandma and grinned. The piano began and Lucy's sweet voice filled the Church. Katie thought she would burst with pride, while holding her breath in case Lucy faltered. She need not have worried, Lucy was looking straight at Joan and singing just like in her living room. She had almost finished; the choir were ready to join in the chorus when realisation hit Katie like a brick. She grabbed Joan's arm and hissed…

Too late!

"Dance Lord wherever you may be, I am the Lord of the dance said he!" trilled Joan in her slightly off-key soprano, drowning out the choir. Lucy looked panicked. She tried to carry on, but it was all going wrong. Why was Grandma singing? She was only supposed to do the grown-up hymns. She looked at her mummy who was pulling at Grandma's sleeve and trying to get her to stop. Joan was oblivious, singing and smiling without a care in the world. There were a few sniggers from behind them. Katie didn't dare turn around. At last, the chorus ended, the teacher indicated the children to sit down and the Headmistress rose to thank everyone for coming before the final prayer. As she bowed her head to pray Katie wasn't sure what to ask for, a quick escape route, a chance to cuddle her clearly distressed child or a quick murderous end to her mother! Then the Head's words pierced her thoughts.

"Finally, a special thank you to Lucy's grandma who worked so hard to help Lucy prepare for her song. Musical talent clearly runs in the family." With a sympathetic glance at Katie, the Head led the children out. Lucy looked a little mollified and at least the sniggers had stopped. Katie helped a beaming Joan to her feet, forgetting the skirt which slipped alarmingly. Not stopping to greet anyone she hurried out of the Church.

"Aren't we staying for cake?" There were refreshments for parents in the Church Hall and Joan was hungry.

"Er, no Mum, sorry I have a lot to do."

*

It was bedtime. Lucy was tired. All day grown-ups had told her how beautifully she had sung. Then other children had made jokes about her stupid grandma. At first, she had been upset by them but in the end she got angry and shouted back at them that her grandma was kind not stupid. That was the truth and after all Grandma had taught her the song. Yet she shouldn't have joined in like that. Her class teacher had told her not to let it spoil her day and had told the class to stop upsetting Lucy. Then she had made this whole speech about old people and being kind. Lucy hadn't really understood it, although at least the teasing stopped. Except from Kai and he was always mean anyway and never did what the teachers told him to do, so he didn't matter.

"Mummy, why did Grandma sing like that?"

Katie looked at Lucy and thought carefully before she answered. "Well, you know how Grandma forgets things lately. Like she always says her telly isn't working when it is and she's just forgotten how to turn it on?"

Lucy nodded not really sure what telly had to do with singing.

"Well, I think Grandma had enjoyed practicing with you so much she just forgot we were in the Church and she wasn't supposed to join in anymore."

Lucy nodded again.

"I'm sorry sweetheart I wouldn't have brought her if I had thought she would spoil it. You sang your part beautifully, I'm very proud of you." She hesitated and then continued, "Grandma is getting old and we might not have her around forever. Maybe we could remember this as a happy time when you sang together? She did enjoy herself so very much. Especially all the practices."

Lucy smiled and nodded gravely. "It was fun singing with Grandma. Though she still shouldn't have sung in Church. It's OK now, my teacher said she was getting very old too and we should be kind and she stopped the others being mean about it."

Katie shuddered inwardly. She hadn't thought about repercussions from other children. Poor Lucy. She said nothing more, simply kissed the top of her head and tucked her under the covers.

Lucy closed her eyes and turned over. She was so very tired; she would think about it all again tomorrow.

77

Chapter 16

Chaos

April 2019

Jack was snoring. Katie stared at the ceiling and sighed. She had two choices. She could poke him, in which case he would wake up, grumble at her but hopefully turn over and sleep more quietly. Or she could leave him be and accept she would get no rest until he turned over naturally. The problem with waking him was that sometimes he took ages to settle back down and blamed her in the morning for his bad night. She didn't want to risk that. She had too much to do. Then again, she needed some sleep. The night wore on, with Jack blissfully snoring and Katie's mind whirring incessantly.

It wasn't just Jack keeping her awake. She was concerned about her mother. The erratic behaviour was getting more extreme. She had found cornflakes in Trixie's bowl again. Her mother had dismissed her concerns with a wave of her hand and an imperious, "I know what my dog likes," comment. Her mother had clearly worn the same clothes for the last three days at least and yet Katie could find nothing dirty in the laundry basket. Not even underwear. Again, this was dismissed as: "I rinse my knickers out in the sink every night". Yet there was none drying anywhere, even if Katie was there before Joan was up. As for food: vegetables rotted in the bottom of the fridge, milk went off, while biscuits and ice cream abounded. Something was seriously wrong and Katie didn't know where to start trying to fix it. Her routine had collapsed under the weight of so many things and she was too busy rushing back and forth dealing with imaginary problems with her mother's TV. Routines just didn't work when so much in her life was unpredictable.

Then there were the children. They had had a peaceful Easter break but now school had restarted and everything was piling up. Matt was happy enough at his new school, although she wasn't sure how much homework he should be doing or even if he did any. He always dismissed her concerns with "I did it in school". That is if he did anything more than grunt at her. She knew he was growing up; she just wasn't ready for teenage angst yet. He was only just 12. Yet the spots were starting, he was shooting up and the grunting…that was very teenage.

She sighed, trying to block out Jack's noise and focus on her daughters. They were OK, weren't they? Molly was so quiet these days. Lucy blew hot and cold. She just didn't have time to sit and listen to her childish babble. Yet sometimes she knew she missed the big stuff…

She turned over, bashed her pillow and tried to block it all out. No sleep would make everything even worse. And she had to work the next day. Starting with the mad rush to deliver the children to breakfast clubs before dashing across town to her school. And bother, she hadn't finished marking the spelling books from last week. She would have to get that done during their quiet reading time. That would mean listening to readers at break to catch up, so no time to phone and check in on Joan. Which would mean a lunch hour of listening to endless messages asking where she was. And she had sewing club at lunch…

She gave up and poked Jack. If she couldn't sleep nor should he!

"Oi what's that for! I was asleep!"

"You were snoring too loud. Just turn over, won't you?"

"I'm awake now! I'll have to go to the loo." Jack stomped off to the ensuite, clearly unhappy at her tactics. She pretended to sleep when he returned but he was determined to have a good long moan. She glanced at the clock; 2.00am. Would she ever get any sleep?

"Mum! Mum! Where are my footy boots?"

"I don't know, where did you last have them?"

"You made me leave them outside last night as they were dirty."

Katie's heart sank.

"Yes- you were supposed to let them dry off and then clean them, did you forget?"

"I had homework!"

"Really?"

"Yes! Maths and chemistry."

"Hmmm…and which of those involved the TV?"

"Everyone needs a break. My teacher says that. Anyway, no sweat my boots will still be by the back door where I left them."

Clearly, he hadn't looked out of the window like Katie had. She inwardly counted to 10 knowing there would be a yell.

"Mum! They're soaking wet!"

By lunchtime Katie was frazzled. Her class had refused to settle into anything after wet play. She knew that was par for the course when children couldn't get outside at break time. However, she was behind on so many things and just needed to get them focussed for five minutes so she could think what to do next. She knew her planning was slipping, her marking was behind and she was not hearing enough readers each day. Yet her mother kept drifting into her mind blocking out all reasonable thought. She was going to have to ring the doctor and see if he would speed up the memory clinic. Surely, they had waited long enough.

Just as she was reaching for her phone to call the doctors an imperious voice cut through her thoughts:

"Does anyone know why the foundation children are outside without their coats on?"

She looked up instantly to see a rather cross looking lunchtime supervisor surrounded by members of her class, looking wet and bedraggled. She realised in a panic she had not checked each child had their coat with them before sending them to lunch. She was used to teaching older children who would know to go back for their coat if they hadn't followed instructions to take it with them to the dining hall. She was still getting used to these little ones who needed spoon feeding every step of the way. She took a deep breath and smiled at the children.

"Come along then let's get back to class and change your school jumpers for your PE ones Then you can stay in with me and play with some of the construction toys."

"You will get a few mums complaining if they go home with wet cardis," muttered the supervisor.

"I will dry them on the radiators, they will be able to put them on again soon. Besides it is only a few drops, or they wouldn't have been outside."

"Should have had their coats on still." The supervisor turned on her heel and went back to her duties.

Katie ushered her charges back into her classroom. No chance of that phone call now.

By the time Katie had seen off the last of her class; dressed back in their dried-out cardigans, tidied her classroom and left notes for her job share it was getting close to 4pm. She had plenty of time to collect the girls by 4.30 and then drive over to Matt's school to collect him from football training. She had a casserole cooking in her slow cooker for dinner, so she felt her tough professional day was going to be counter balanced by a well organised evening. She checked her phone as she walked to her car. Joan's plaintive voice was repeatedly on voicemail. Her heating wasn't working and she was cold.

"Darn it!" she said out loud as she started to calculate her best route. Grab the girls, squeeze in checking on Joan and then be a little late for Matt, or collect him a bit early and then do Mum? Neither was very feasible and both would draw loud protests from Matt and probably the girls too. Still, she couldn't leave her mum sitting in the cold. Yet she had no idea how to fix heating problems. This was going to involve calling out a plumber and lots of waiting around. She decided on a novel but probably best chance of success approach. She would collect the children as usual, take them home and serve their dinner. Then when Jack got home, she would slip off to her mother's house. She knew Jack would be unhappy, although even he would not expect her mum to sit in the cold. She also thought she would cut waiting time and call the plumbers in advance from her house. She rang Joan to reassure her she would be over soon and suggest she put an extra jumper on for now. While Joan sounded confused and frightened, she accepted Katie's plan and promised to wrap up until she arrived.

Naturally Jack was late home. Last minute meeting was all he said, startled at Katie's impatience when he sloped through the door just before 7.00. She had little time to explain anything as the plumber had told her he would arrive around 7.30 and she was worried Joan might turn him away. Lucy was ready for bed and the older two were watching TV, homework presumably done. All Jack needed to do was tuck Lucy in and remind the others to go up to bed on time. His dinner was in the microwave and all the dishes were done. Jack scowled but made no attempt to stop her escape.

As Katie backed out of the drive, she rubbed her eyes. She was so tired. All she wanted was a hot soak and an early night. However, she couldn't leave her mum in the cold.

"Hello? Mum! Where are you?" Katie called out to Joan as she opened the door.

"I'm here dear, a nice gentleman is here to mend my boiler." Momentary panic that she was late was replaced by concern for the cost if it was the boiler at fault. A short, dark-haired man with a protruding belly hanging over his low-slung waistband appeared from the cupboard under the stairs.

"Was it you who called me out?"

"Er yes I'm Joan's daughter Katie, I thought I would be here before you arrived."

"Only been here a minute so you're OK and your mum makes a nice cuppa."

"So, what seems to be the problem?" The man shifted slightly, before nodding towards the kitchen.

"I reckon as your daughter might like one of those cuppa's Joan."

Katie was startled by the comment, then something in his eyes made her smile and nod, "Yes please Mum."

"There's nothing wrong with the boiler, or the radiators or any part of the system you will be pleased to know. But there is a problem. Your mum has been turning the boiler off at night. She told me it is very noisy and keeps her awake. Trouble is a system like this shouldn't be switched off at the mains like that too often. It makes the pilot light go out which is what happened here. Then the safety all kicks in and nothing will start up. All she needs to do is turn the thermostat down to reduce the heat or even stop the noise. Not that there is any real noise. Silent running this system, just a sound when it starts up. Not my place to say this really but she doesn't seem to understand what I'm telling her and…" he shifted uncomfortably, "…well it is going to keep happening if she won't change her ways…and I do have to charge you for the call out."

"I understand. I'll try to explain to her what you have told me."

The man bent down to pack up his tools, exposing more of his rear end than Katie really wanted to see. He straightened up, fixed Katie with a sympathetic smile which came across as more of a grimace and added. "My mum was the same, started doing odd things, ended up in a home. Not my place to give advice, but I think your mum needs some help."

"Thank you," said Katie more firmly than she had intended, then continued "I do as much as I can, but I have three children and a job." She couldn't understand quite why she was excusing herself to the plumber, even if his concern seemed genuine.

"My missus tried too, but in the end it was too much. Well, that's all I can say really. Now will you pay cash or BACS?"

After paying the plumber Katie sat with Joan a while as the heating kicked in. Once she was sure her mum was warm and comfortable, she felt ready to go home. She couldn't leave without one more attempt at making sure her mum didn't turn the boiler off again though.

"Right Mum, now you heard what the man said. You must not turn off the main switch. Just turn down the thermostat if it gets too hot or too erm noisy and everything will work just fine."

Joan stared at her belligerently. "I have to turn it off, it keeps me awake!"

"Mum, as the plumber said, you will break the system. Listen it isn't making any noise now."

"You aren't in my bedroom! That's where the problem is."

"OK Mum let's go and see."

Katie stood in her mother's room and listened. No sound could be heard except a few cars outside. The boiler was silent.

"It starts up later. Keeps me awake for hours."

"If you turn it off it won't come back on and you will be cold Mum."

"It comes on fine in the mornings I just press the switch."

"Yes, it does most mornings but over time it won't. And then like today you will be cold all day."

"I'll just put an extra jumper on and wait for that nice plumber to come again then." Katie's insides knotted at Joan's bright enthusiasm. She tried and failed to keep the frustration from her voice.

"Mum that nice plumber cost £50. He can't keep coming over just because you won't do the right thing."

"Don't speak to me like that Katie! I'm still your mother!"

Katie felt weak. It had been such a long difficult day, tears threatened and she just wanted to go home. Instead, she summoned her most patient "dealing with a small child" voice.

"Well Mum, I have to go home now. The heating is on. I have set the timer so it will turn off by 10.00 and come back on in the morning. You get yourself into bed and try to sleep. The clever man fixed the noise so that is all gone. Listen- nothing! Wasn't he clever! And he loved your tea."

Joan stared quizzically at Katie as if not quite understanding this new approach. "He fixed the noise?"

"Yes totally. It's gone for ever."

"We'll see," muttered Joan darkly, although she looked calmer. Katie gave her a kiss and started to go downstairs. When she reached the front door, she saw her sign reminding her mum to take her keys. In a flash of inspiration, she hurried back into the kitchen and scrabbled to find pen, paper and Sellotape. She wrote "DO NOT TURN OFF." In big black letters and stuck it over the main boiler switch. Hopefully that would work.

She slipped out of the door and turned thankfully for home. With luck all three children would be in bed and she could quickly follow them. Hopefully Jack would not snore tonight…

Chapter 17

After Chaos

April 2019

It was dark. Was it still night or were the curtains just blocking out the light? Joan pulled herself upright and blinked. She stared around her wondering for a moment where she was. She could hear loud insistent barking from somewhere. Really people should keep their dogs quiet at night. She thought carefully. Was she still tired? She decided she was and lay back down.

When she woke again, she was sure it was morning as light was pushing itself around the curtains. She stretched and looked around for some clothes. There was a pile on her chair, so she put them on. Then she went through to the bathroom and washed her face and combed her hair. She realised she was hungry. She went downstairs. Trixie was waiting in the kitchen, tail wagging furiously. For a moment Joan wondered whose dog it was and then laughed at herself.

"Silly me! Good morning Trixie, shall I let you out?" she opened the door and Trixie bounded gratefully outside. She closed the door.

Breakfast! She opened her cupboards one by one until she found a bowl, some cornflakes and a bag of sugar. She took a spoon from the drawer and heaped sugar onto the cereal. She looked round for the fridge. Trixie was by now scraping at the door to come in, but unable to place the noise Joan ignored her. Instead, she stared at the contents of her fridge. No milk! Sighing she closed the door and went into the hall to find her coat and shoes. It took her a while to locate her handbag before she opened the front door. At the last minute she responded to Katie's door sign and remembered to take her keys. Closing the front door, she set off to the nearby co-op.

"Hello Mrs Jessup, how are you today?" A total stranger was smiling at her. She smiled back.

"Fine thank you."

"Weather's not too bad today is it? For this time of year."

"No, it's quite pleasant." Her neighbour nodded and continued her shopping.

Joan looked around. What was it she needed? She knew she was hungry. She looked at the large clock on the wall. Eleven O'clock.

"Ah elevenses!" She smiled to herself. What to have? Jaffa cakes were on offer or there were some lovely little iced buns. She chose the buns and put them carefully in her basket. Then she added the Jaffa cakes for later.

"Is that all?" The young shop assistant barely looked up as she emptied Joan's basket.

"Er… no I'll have one of these!" Joan added a Kit Kat from the display in front of the counter.

"Treating yourself a bit!" It was the stranger again.

"Well yes I thought I'd have something nice for when Katie comes."

"Oh that's lovely. Will she bring the children?"

"Oh yes she always does."

"That's nice. As you know my children live too far away for me to see them very often. You are so lucky."

"Yes I am," beamed Joan

"That's £4.22 please." The assistant cut across the conversation.

"Oh yes, let's see." Joan scrabbled in her purse looking for the right money.

"Just give me the fiver I've got change."

"Oh no I'm nearly there. That's it! £ 3.24!"

"Its £4.22 you need."

"Oh...I think I can make another pound. Yes...a fifty, two tens, a twenty and here's two five pence. "

The assistant made a show of carefully counting each coin before wordlessly handing Joan back two pence.

"Thank you!" Joan beamed again and hurried off with her goodies. She let herself into her house and looked around for the dog. How odd that she wasn't there. Worried she hurried through the kitchen and opened the back door. There was Trixie wagging her tail.

"How ever did you get out there? Come on in silly dog!" Joan sat down to eat her goodies. Trixie barked.

"Oh you can't have these, they aren't for dogs." Trixie barked again. Joan looked around and saw the bowl of sugar laden cornflakes.

"There you didn't eat your breakfast! Here you go!" Trixie sniffed, whined, ate a couple of mouthfuls in desperation and then slunk miserably back to her bed. Joan tucked into her buns.

Chapter 18

Scammers

April 2019

Some days still went swimmingly. Katie would drop the children at the school, then pop into her mum's house for a coffee and a chat. Inevitably there would be some household tasks to do, although she made sure she managed to escape in time to grab some lunch before starting on her own chores. Even some workdays went smoothly. Again, she would drop the children off, dash breathlessly into work, turn off her phone and zip it into the deepest recesses of her handbag before focussing on the children in front of her. She loved teaching. The more she did it the more she blossomed in the environment. She celebrated every little achievement for every child. She found herself drawn more and more to those who struggled and started to contemplate some training to specialise in learning support. That was when she was living a good day and fantasising about her future career. On the bad days she could see nothing but black exhaustion and swirling chaos. Determinedly, she pushed those ruthlessly aside as though she could stop the descent by sheer will power and forge ahead.

"Mum! I need my footie kit!"

"Mum! Can I go to Jamie's for tea tomorrow?"

"Mummy! I can't find my reading book!"

"Katie, I said I needed a blue shirt today for my presentation."

"It's in your PE bag in the laundry room, yes I'll speak to her mum today to make arrangements and I think you put it back in your book bag last night. And that one is blue."

"I wanted light blue. To go with my tie."

"I thought modern business dress meant no ties."

'Seriously Kate don't be glib. Is there a light blue one anywhere?"

"In the wash probably. You will have to choose another tie. C'mon girls let's get in the car. Matt your bus leaves in two minutes!"

Grabbing her keys and ignoring Jack's muttering, she ushered the girls out of the door. As she reached the car, she heard a persistent ringing. Ignoring her phone, she strapped in Lucy, settled herself and pulled out of the drive. The phone rang again.

"Molly, can you answer that? It's in the front of my bag. Tell Grandma I'm driving and will be at work today. I will call her lunchtime."

She listened as Molly relayed the message.

"Mum…I think you need to go to Grandma's."

"I can't I have to go to work."

'She sounded really upset."

"I know Molly she always does. Unfortunately, she is getting very forgetful and it scares her sometimes. Don't worry. If I've time I will ring her as soon as I get to school before the children arrive."

'She said she needs your help."

"Did she say why."

"No just that she needs you to go there quickly."

'Sweetheart I know it sounds real, but it is usually just that she can't find the remote or remember where she left her cup of tea. I promise you it will be nothing. Look, here we are at drop off. You take Lucy into breakfast club for me and I will be able to make time to ring Grandma as soon as I reach school."

However, when she reached school, the deputy needed a chat before the staff briefing. Then before she knew it the children were piling in and she was caught up in the day's events. Lunchtime was taken up with her sewing club, the afternoon was full of changing for PE and back again as well as teaching, followed by frantically marking her books before rushing to get the girls.

"Did you speak to Grandma? Was she OK?" Molly's voice quavered. Clearly, she had thought more about it than Kate had. Pushing aside her guilt Katie made a mental note to turn off her phone before they got in the car and not let Molly use it anymore. It had worked so many times. Molly and Joan had had a lovely cosy chat as Katie drove and Joan's need for company had been eased.

"Erm…'she bit her lip not wanting to lie, while hating the anxiety on Molly's face.

"Tell you what, why don't we pop in on the way home? You can take Trixie for a little walk down the lane if you like. She would love that. And you can see for yourself Grandma is fine."

"Can I go too?"

"You are a bit little still Lucy. You can play ball with Trixie when they get back." Lucy stuck her bottom lip out but didn't protest. Katie turned for her mother's, silently re-planning a quicker evening meal in her head.

As she turned into her mother's drive, she noticed how tidy the garden looked. Her mother had ignored the autumn leaves when they fell, saying they would rot down in time for Spring. Well it was Spring now and she had clearly spent a lot of time sweeping leaves today. Either that or the good fairy had been again. She was still bemused by the things her mum said "Katy did" when she knew she hadn't.

"Hello Mum! We thought we would pop in to see how you are. Molly wants to walk the dog and Lucy is going to play ball with her."

"That's nice."

As Molly put the excited little dog on her lead and Lucy searched for a ball, Katie looked around her. Clearly the good fairy hadn't been in the house.

"How have you been Mum? I'm sorry I haven't rung. It was a school day." Katie filled the kettle as Molly slipped out the door.

"Don't go out of the street!"

"I won't Mum, just to the corner and back."

"Oh I haven't done much. Watched a bit of telly."

"What about your garden Mum. Did you rake all those leaves?"

"Oh…no…the gardeners did it. The ones you sent."

"I didn't send any gardeners Mum."

"Oh…well they were very good. It's all tidy now."

"Did you pay them Mum?"

"Of course!"

"How much."

Joan frowned.

"Mum…?"

"There was a bit of a fuss. I didn't have enough. So we went to the co-op. But a policeman came and the gardeners left."

"What!"

"Don't worry Katie it's not important."

"Of course…"

Her phone rang. As she glanced to check the number, she saw 7 missed calls.

"Let me just answer this Mum then we will talk more."

"Hello?"

"This is PC Talbot. Is that Mrs Robinson?"

"Yes. Is this about my mother? I'm with her now."

"Yes. I think she has been a victim of a fraud. Do you think I could come to meet you? Your Mum doesn't seem to have a clear grasp of what happened."

"Yes, please absolutely. "

"I will be there in half an hour."

"Thank you."

"Mummy! Molly won't let me have a turn with the ball!"

"Oh never mind Lucy."

"But it's not fair she went for the walk."

"Molly give her a go please."

"I did but she can't throw it far enough and Trixie doesn't like it."

"I'm hungry Mummy."

"Just go and play nicely with the dog girls, I need to talk to Daddy." Recognising the seriousness in her mother's voice Molly ushered hungry Lucy away. Meanwhile Joan stared at her daughter, a look of defiance on her face.

"Jack it's me. I'm at Mum's."

"Typical. So no dinner for me I suppose, honestly Katie it is not good enough I…"

'Shut up and listen for once, the police are on their way. Mum has been scammed. I need you to get home on time, feed Matt and then come here and collect the girls. No actually, change that around, collect the girls on your way. I will text Matt and tell him you are coming. He can have a sandwich while he waits. There's plenty of left-over roast and some salad so you will all be fine. Molly will help you put it on a plate and serve."

"You expect me to just need to drop everything and come running."

"Please."

"I can't leave till 5.30 I have meetings."

"I don't want the girls exposed to this. Police and everything. Especially Lucy. And it might take ages."

"I jolly well hope not!"

"Can you come." She felt the pause at the other end of the line, hoping that for once Jack might actually help."

"OK, give me time to shuffle a few things round. I should be with you in half an hour."

"Thank you."

"Mum! Lucy fell over!" Quickly Katie hung up and rushed to assess the damage. Just a minor scrape. She washed the cut and settled the girls with juice and biscuits in front of the TV.

"Right Mum let's go in the kitchen and put the kettle on and you can tell me a bit more about the gardeners."

Jack arrived just seconds before the policeman. He ushered an anxious Molly and a grumpy Lucy into the car, pausing only to check Katie was OK to handle things before driving off. Katie hoped the children would cooperate although she had no time to think about it much, as PC Talbot pulled up with a lady policewoman beside him.

"Good afternoon I'm PC Talbot and this is PC Kumar."

"Come on in, Mum is in here."

"Hello again Mrs Jessup how are you feeling now?"

Joan frowned, "Have we met?"

"Earlier today at the Co-op, remember?"

"Oh yes of course."

So far, all Katie had ascertained was that the 'gardeners' had asked for more money than Joan had and so they had taken her to a cash point. Joan had never used one so instead she went into the Co-op to get cash back which was her usual practice. For some reason then the police had intervened. Joan had not been happy and couldn't understand all the fuss.

PC Talbot gave more details.

"Your mother was asked by some gentlemen, who we have been monitoring for some time, if she wanted her leaves cleared. Obviously, we were not party to that conversation, but their usual practice is to quote a reasonable price; £20 for instance. Then when the work is done, they ask for £200. It is rare that older people have that kind of money on them, so they insist on going to a cash point to take it out. As your mother couldn't get cash from the machine, they went with her into the shop to get cash back. Thankfully the shop only allows £50 per transaction and when your mum went around a second time to get just a tin of beans, the staff were concerned. They saw the men hanging around watching and decided to call us. When we pulled up the men vanished of course. I believe your mum had paid them £100 by then."

"Oh Mum is that true?"

"I owed them money; they did the work."

"Raking a few leaves up isn't worth that much!"

"Then why did you send them?"

"I didn't."

"I phoned you to check."

"Oh Mum I was at work- look," she showed her mother her phone with all the missed calls. I would have told you and written it on your board if I had sent them."

"What happens now?" Katie turned back to the police.

"There is a chance they will come back in the next few days to demand the rest. Try to make sure your mother isn't alone, or that she doesn't open the door to anyone. I would also appreciate it if you could do an online fraud report. The more of these we have the better chance we have of a conviction."

"Can't you arrest them now?"

'Sadly no, as we have no evidence. They only pick on the elderly. Most of those who fall for it have, erm, memory lapses. We are building up a dossier and hopefully in time we will have enough."

"And we can't get Mum's money back?"

"I don't want it back I paid them to do a job!" Joan interjected defiantly, "You are all making too much of this! They were very nice men."

"We understand that this is confusing Mrs Jessup, but those men were stealing from you. Please don't let them in again or give them any more money." The policewoman spoke softly yet firmly. Joan glared and said no more.

"I would suggest that you use your power of attorney to freeze your mother's accounts for a few days. Just to make sure nothing else is taken out. Then take a long hard look at how your mother manages her account. You can set a £50 limit per day to help protect her from these kinds of things. Get some advice. The Alzheimer's society are very good."

"Um… OK … It's just I don't actually have a power of attorney set up. And Mum doesn't have a diagnosis of anything yet. We are waiting on an appointment." Katie felt very sheepish as the policeman smiled sympathetically.

"I'm not a doctor obviously, but I would definitely class your mum as vulnerable. All kinds of people prey on the elderly these days. We can come back and do a safety and security check on the house and the fire service will do a fire check. However, I think you may need to look at alternative living arrangements sometime in the not too distant future. If you can that is. Just to keep your mum safe. For now, get that LPA sorted and protect her from scammers. There are a lot of phone scammers out there too that ring the elderly and ask for cash. You can put her number on a register to stop it happening too much, although they find ways around it. As for postal begging letters, it's hard to stop those even with the postal service blocks you can do. Does she use the internet?"

"No."

"Just as well."

"I can leave you some leaflets to explain some of these things. Here's my card so if you need help you can call. I will drive past the house every day this week and keep an eye out for these blokes, but like I said, it's best if your mum isn't alone as much as possible."

Katie swallowed hard and took the leaflets. "Thank you, you have been very kind."

"And get on and sort the LPA. That's my best advice. Quickly."

"Thank you. I will deal with it all." Katie saw the police out then turned to Joan.

'Stuff and nonsense, I'm fine. I will pay whoever I like to do my garden!"

Katie stayed with her mother as long as she dared. However, by 7.00 she felt she needed to go home to tuck Lucy into bed. She put a large notice on the inside of the front door saying, "DO NOT OPEN TO ANYONE EXCEPT FAMILY". And hoped that would dissuade her mother. She intended to be there straight after the school run the next few days and stand guard until pick up time when she would take Joan with her. What she would do on Friday when she had to work, she simply did not know.

She slipped in quietly and was amazed to see Jack sitting in front of the TV. She had expected chaos.

"Lucy's asleep." He said smugly, "and the other two are in their rooms reading."

"How…?"

"We had pizza for tea and I promised them unlimited telly tomorrow after school if they were good tonight."

"Ok…"

"Look it worked, didn't it? Now tell me about this scam and what's to be done."

Katie went through the advice the police had given. Jack was attentive and helpful. He explained how the LPA forms could be found on the internet and easily completed. He offered to organise that for Katie and even suggested he be added as a safeguard. There was no one else. Katie made a list of people to contact to protect her mother's phone and postal ID and other actions the police had suggested. Finally, Jack raised the subject she was avoiding.

"We need to start looking at homes love. Your mum isn't going to get better. This has proved she can't stay there alone indefinitely. And you can't carry on being run ragged by all this."

"She won't like it."

"No…but what other choice is there? She needs to be safe."

Katie bit her lip. "Let's wait till we have a diagnosis. It might not be…"

Jack uncharacteristically said nothing but merely pulled her close. Breathing in his warmth Katie wondered why he was being so kind this time. No complaining, no sulking. Then guiltily she pushed the thought away and sunk into his arms, grateful for the comfort. He had always been good in a real crisis, just not in the little, daily, niggly things. And this was real now. Her mother was struggling and no amount of wishing she wasn't was going to fix it or make it go away. She was going to have to deal with it. Tomorrow I'll think about all this she thought, suddenly overwhelmed with tiredness. Tomorrow will be easier perhaps.

Joan was tired too. She let Trixie out in the garden to relieve herself and then slipped upstairs. The dog could come in when she was ready. It was dark and she needed to go to bed.

Chapter 19

Toads

April 2019

After a couple of days of worry and rushing back and forth to her mother's, Katie decided the best solution was to have Joan stay with them for a few days. Trixie had to go to kennels due to Jack's allergy, which would cost a bit. On the positive side, it gave her a chance to watch her mother up close. It was all going well, although her mother's constant inability to find her own bedroom was alarming. She was sleeping in Molly's room and the girls were squeezed in together. Not ideal but OK as a temporary measure. Besides not having to rush across town every day gave Katie some breathing space. Also, her mother was at least eating better. Today though her mother wasn't the problem.

"I don't want to!" Lucy screwed up her face in disgust and stamped her foot to emphasise the point.

"Oh Lucy don't be so difficult it will only take a minute." Lucy was tired. She had been to school and stayed for her extra maths club and now she was comfortable watching TV. She absolutely did not want to get in the car and go to get Molly from her playdate. She knew mummy would win in the end and make her go as she was a grown up and Lucy was the youngest. Sometimes being the youngest was hard.

"You let Matt stay on his own yesterday." She added." When Molly and I had to come with you to the shops he stayed home all by himself!"

"Lucy, I don't have time for this. Matt is 12 you are 5 and we were only gone a few minutes."

"But I'm nearly 6 and you said we would only be a few minutes to get Molly."

"For the last time Lucy get your shoes on!"

"That's a mean voice and you didn't say please." Katie's sharp intake of breath could be heard three streets away.

"Put your shoes on now- please!"

"I don't want to."

"Lucy you absolutely cannot stay here alone."

"Matt did!"

"Matt is 12 and besides he wasn't alone, Grandma was here."

Lucy's face broke out into an enormous grin.

"Grandma is here now, so I can stay with her!" Katie winced. How could she have been so stupid. It was one thing leaving Matt with her mother for 15 minutes while they whizzed to the shops for some forgotten ingredients for dinner. Leaving her 5 year-old in the care of her mother, that was quite different. How to explain that to Lucy?

"You can't stay with Grandma she's having a nap," she tried lamely.

"I'll just watch TV and I can wake her up if I need her." Lucy was wheedling now. She knew she should just go but her favourite show was about to start and if Grandma was there why couldn't she stay? Grandma had looked after her lots when she was really little.

"It wouldn't be fair to wake Grandma." Katie said firmly." Now come on!"

"I want to stay with Grandma!"

At that moment, to Katie's horror, Joan shuffled into the living room.

"Grandma! Mummy said you were asleep. As you are awake, can I stay with you please, while she goes to get Molly, can I, can I please?"

"Of course you can sweetheart," said Joan, then after seeing Katie's face she added, "If your mum says you can." Katie hesitated. She knew Lucy was tired and would probably stay watching the TV. She was already late and needed to get Molly home and the dinner on in time for Matt to eat before Scouts. She knew her mum was no longer a fit babysitter. Yet to try to explain that to both of them now. There just wasn't time and she didn't have the words.

"OK you can stay, just be really good for Grandma!"

Lucy threw her arms round her mother. "I will Mummy I promise."

With a last worried glance back Katie slipped out the door. She knew she was doing the wrong thing and that she would have to talk to her mum about not babysitting anymore at some point soon. She would only be 15 minutes, or 20 at most. It would be OK today. Just this once.

30 minutes later….

Katie practically ran through the door. There had been a burst water pipe in the road outside Tracey's house causing a jam and she had abandoned the car in a side road and run the last few yards to pick up Molly. Then Tracey's mum had asked about lifts to ballet classes delaying her further. She had hauled a protesting Molly down the road at breakneck pace and driven as fast as she dared. All the time her brain racing with "what ifs".

"Mum! Lucy! We're home!" No one answered.

The TV was still on, although Lucy was not watching it. Katie raced through the house checking every room, calling for them. Molly watched, confused by her mother's obvious panic. The back door was open; they must have gone outside. Molly looked in the garden.

"Are they there?" a breathless Katie grabbed Molly's arms as she came back indoors.

"No Mum." Katie let out a wail. Then seeing the terror on Molly's face, she took a breath. Now be logical. Where could they have gone? The park? The shops? And why?

"We have to go and look for them Molly. Put your shoes back on." Mystified, Molly did as she was told. She didn't understand why her mother was behaving like this. If Grandma and Lucy had gone out together, they would come back. Grandma had always looked after them all. Just as they opened the door to leave, in came Grandma and an exuberant Lucy.

"Where have you been!" snapped Katie.

Joan flinched at the anger in Katie's voice and Lucy's excitement evaporated.

"We found a big toad in the garden," said Joan. The neighbour's dog was barking at it and I thought it might hurt it.

Lucy and I put it in a box and took it to the pond at the end of the lane."

"You were supposed to just watch television!"

Suddenly Lucy felt very small and sad. Her mummy was being horrid today and she didn't think she had done anything bad. She had heard the dog barking and Grandma had gone to investigate. They had thought it would be a good thing to help the toad. It had been hard to catch it using the net from Daddy's fishing set. She was proud they had done it and now the toad was safe by the pond. Mummy always told them to be kind to animals so why was she so cross? Lucy had even missed her favourite show to do it! With as much dignity as she could muster in her 5-year-old frame she turned on her heels and with a last look at her mother, stomped off upstairs. She paused as she got to the top.

"Thank you Grandma for a nice time. I'm glad we saved the toad." Joan stared at Katie. She couldn't understand any of this. She had thoroughly enjoyed being with Lucy. Katie must just be tired. She worked too hard.

"Shall I make us a cup of tea?"

"I need to start the dinner." Katie snapped back. She knew she was being unfair. Why was this all so hard?

"I'm sorry Mum. We'll talk later." Joan's bewildered stare left Katie wretched. Right now, she had to make dinner. It would all have to wait. Later they would talk. She would find the words to explain. Just not now, not till her heart returned to normal and she could let out the terror that had drenched her. Not till then. Later. She would deal with it all later.

Chapter 20

Clean Houses

April 2019

Katie rubbed her eyes. She was sitting at the school gates after dropping off the girls. Molly had taken to walking Lucy to her class before going to her own. Katie would sit and watch her daughters until they disappeared. It was kind of Molly, but it made her feel curiously detached from the school. As an only child she was never sure about sibling dynamics. She just knew it made life a little easier as she could watch from the drop off zone rather than having to find a place to park.

She felt furious with herself for treating Lucy so badly over the toad. She knew she had been unnecessarily harsh. Molly bothered her too. She crept around the house like a shadow, making no sound unless forced. Matt on the other hand was becoming louder and more unruly by the minute. She felt she was losing touch with all her children and yet had no idea how to stop the decline. Or perhaps she did, but she just didn't want to do it. Should she give up her job like Jack wanted?

That morning, as always when something at home wasn't perfect, Jack had gone on the attack. Katie had forgotten he had a special presentation to do and so his best shirt had not been washed. Her job he had stated firmly was to support him in all he did and make sure his home ran smoothly. Such antiquated ideas belonged in the 19th century she had countered. And yet…that had been their agreement. She had wanted more children. He had needed to work long, hard hours to take care of them all. Her little part time insignificant salary made no real contribution to their budget. Was life only about money? She loved her job, loved the way it made her feel useful in a way that ironing perfect shirts never had.

And then of course there was Mum. Perhaps her return to work would have gone better if it hadn't coincided with her mother's decline. She knew she couldn't abandon her mother. There was no one else who would step in. Joan had moved back home after the toad episode and she needed to get over there as quickly as she could now, to ensure she could get back in time to make sure her home was ship shape. Then she would make one of Jack's favourite dinners, something she could prepare early to enable her to spend some time with each of the children when they got in from school. Then maybe they could even play a game all together like they used to after dinner. What was the name of that board game they all loved? Frustration. That was it. Katie started to laugh. How appropriate was that!

When she reached Joan's house all was quiet and the curtains were still drawn. Katie let herself in. Trixie greeted her furiously, tail wagging with excitement. She let the little dog out into the garden and filled her food and water bowls. She crept upstairs to peek in on Joan. Sound asleep. She grabbed the washing basket and any items dropped around the bed and bathroom and filled the machine. Then she set to scrubbing, tidying and polishing the little house until everything gleamed. She didn't get the hoover out until last. She hadn't wanted to wake her mother until she was done, as Joan would always fret that Katie was cleaning for her. Joan seemed to think the house never got dirty anymore. Yet without Katie's weekly deep clean it would be a health hazard. Joan had taken to sleeping all morning lately, which meant Katie could be done before she woke.

Trixie stared at her hopefully, tail thumping madly. She needed a walk. Perhaps Katie could even do that before Joan woke?

"Who's there? Who's in my house? I have a dog you know!" Joan's feeble voice sounded down the stairs.

"It's only me Mum."

"Oh Katie you scared me! Why are you here in the middle of the night?"

"It's morning Mum. I just popped in to see you. Would you like a nice cup of tea up there?"

"Urm yes of course it is, I hadn't looked out the window yet. Yes, tea would be lovely thank you."

Katie quickly brewed the tea and added a bowl of cereal to her mum's tray. She smiled as she set it down by Joan's bed.

"You have some breakfast in bed Mum and I'll run you a bath."

"You don't need to do that!"

"I want to spoil you Mum. I've got some lovely smelly bubbles to put in." Katie suspected her mother no longer bathed unless she was encouraged to. She couldn't comprehend the changes in her mother. She had always been so particular. If only that doctor's referral would come through. They might get to the bottom of the problem. Katie pushed her thoughts of diagnosis aside. She was not going to guess at anything. Just wait for the specialist.

While Joan bathed, Katie whipped the hoover round and made the bed. She laid out some nice clean clothes for her mother.

"It's a lovely day out Mum shall we walk Trixie together once you are up?"

"That would be lovely. Do you have time."

Katie looked at the little dog's hopeful brown eyes. "Of course I do Mum."

On the way home, after leaving her mum both a meal for lunch and a sandwich in the fridge for tea, she felt successful. She had at least got her mother's house in order. She had a new system planned now. On all her days off she would go straight there from school drop off. Once a week to clean, once to deliver shopping that she would add to her own supermarket delivery the day before. She couldn't imagine why she hadn't thought of having a delivery before. So much easier than pushing a trolley around and all that lifting heavy bags. On the third day she would simply visit. She could make sure her mother ate properly on those days and Trixie was walked and fed. On the days she worked she could only phone. The hardest days would be weekends. However, despite Jack's disapproval she intended to call in at least one of the days. She felt then she could get a little bit on top of things. She knew her own home was looking neglected and her washing pile grew ever larger. However, her priorities needed to be that her mother was safe and that she found time for each of her children. A little bit of dirt in the house didn't matter so much. Full of resolve she pulled into her drive.

She turned the key in the lock of her front door. As she opened it the smell of unwashed breakfast dishes assailed her. She glanced around critically. Her home looked unkempt and unloved. Was this what Jack saw when he came through the door? She rolled up her sleeves and started again.

Later falling asleep in front of Jack's favourite TV show, Katie ruminated about the evening. The meal had been lovely, with even Molly joining in the conversation. They had struggled through a game of Monopoly, as apparently Frustration was for babies. Katie and Lucy had worked as a team. Matt had insisted on being banker and Jack had been impatient with his slow money management, yet all in all they had negotiated it quite well. She had done it. A successful family day…

"Thank you."

"For what?"

"For remembering your role. Life does only go smoothly when we all play our part you know. It was lovely coming home to a clean efficient house once more. Do think again about that job of yours. It would be so good to get back to normal."

Too tired to respond Katie turned her head and let her tears slip silently onto the pillow.

Chapter 21

Diagnosis

May 2019

Katie was tired. So tired her bones ached. She longed to ignore the alarm and just roll over. But Jack was already up and dressing and she could hear Lucy clattering about in her room. She forced her eyes open and glanced at her phone to check appointments. Then the cold fist settled back in her stomach as she remembered, today was the day of the test.

"Come on Lucy!" She tried in vain each morning to get Lucy to dress herself. Somehow it always ended with her sitting on the bed squeezing her wriggling, squirming child into her clothes. She knew she should be firmer. Lucy was always in trouble at school for taking too long to change for PE. It remained one of those things she would get around to when everything else was sorted. Whenever that might be.

"My tummy hurts," said Lucy.

Automatically Katie felt Lucy's forehead. It felt normal.

"I'm sure you are fine." she said, her mind on her mother.

"But it hurts!" said Lucy insistently, "I can't go to school!"

Katie stared at her daughter. It had taken months for this memory clinic appointment to come through. Months where her mother's confusion had deepened and the chaos it created in Katie's life had swirled ever wilder. Lucy could not be sick today. Not when the solution was at hand.

"Maybe you are just hungry. Perhaps some breakfast would help." Lucy's little face scrunched up.

"I'm not hungry, my tummy hurts!"

"You can have coco pops."

"You never let me have coco pops. You said you threw them away." Suspicion etched firmly into Lucy's face.

On the one and only occasion Jack had offered to do the weekly shop he had inexplicably come home with the offending cereal. Katie never allowed her children such a sugar rush at breakfast. Jack had shrugged and said he fancied them as they reminded him of his childhood. Once Katie had finished unpacking all the other sweet sugary rubbish that he had bought, she had vowed never to let him return unaccompanied to the shops. Naturally he had taken that as his cue not to help again. The children however had been hugely excited at the idea of chocolate cereal. After one nightmare Saturday of sugar fuelled frenzy, Katie had shoved it to the back of the cupboard for Jack to retrieve if he ever wanted to revisit his malnourished upbringing and told them it was in the bin.

Now she was offering it as a bribe to get Lucy to school.

She shook the sensible notion that a sick child needed a light healthy breakfast from her head, as Lucy slowly followed her downstairs and watched in disbelief while her mother poured coco pops into her bowl, smothered them with milk and placed them on the table.

Lucy took one spoonful, then another, coughed slightly and then threw up a brown slushy mess speckled with undigested, crushed, brown pops.

Katie tried to ignore the rising panic as she ushered Lucy back upstairs, cleaned her up and tucked her back into bed. There was only one answer.

"Try to sleep sweetheart, Mummy has to take Grandma to the doctor, so Daddy will look after you."

"Don't be silly Mummy, Daddy goes to work!"

"Not today."

Rushing back downstairs she saw Molly packing her bag. "We're leaving in one minute. Be ready," she hissed, ignoring Molly's startled face. She grabbed a pen and pad and scribbled instructions.

Jack was folding his newspaper and tucking it into his briefcase. She squared her shoulders, imagined she was facing her class at school and spoke.

"Today is the day of Mum's memory clinic appointment. Unfortunately, Lucy is sick and needs to stay in bed. You will have to look after her. I've written a list of suggestions, what to look out for and when you might need to call a doctor. His number is there too. I'm sure you'll cope."

Jack just starred.

"You'll have to ring the office and tell them you can't come in."

"Don't be ridiculous!"

Molly appeared behind Katie, coat and shoes on, bag in hand.

"I have waited months for this Jack, I'm taking Molly to school now and then I will be taking Mum. Look after Lucy she has a stomach ache and has been sick. Plenty of fluids no food."

Then with a last glance at the congealing vomit on the kitchen table, she pushed past Jack, pulling an astonished Molly behind her and exited.

Jack followed her out protesting loudly that children need their mothers when they are sick, he needed to be at a meeting and this was just typically selfish behaviour putting her mother above them all. Katie blanked out his stream of words as she dragged Molly down the drive. Jack was still yelling for her to come back at once, as she pushed Molly into the car and whizzed away.

After dropping a bemused Molly at school, Katie drove carefully across town to her mother's house. The curtains were drawn and no lights on. She knocked at the door, but no one answered, although the dog barked loudly. She opened the door with her key. The dog leapt at her licking her face. Sheets of newspaper flapped around and a strong smell of urine rose from the carpet. Switching on the hall light Katie called out to her mum. No answer. She went through to the kitchen. No sign of Joan. The dog's water and food bowls were empty and last night's attempt at dinner sat half eaten on the table with various mugs of half-drunk tea scattered around the room. Dirty dishes and saucepans with baked on grime were piled in the sink. It had only been two days since Katie's last visit. She wrinkled her nose at the pungent smells, then spotted a pile of faeces in the corner by the back door, where the dog was now frantically scraping and barking. She let her out and turned to go upstairs in search of her mother.

"Hello love what a nice surprise!" Joan materialised in the hallway, still in her night gown, obviously just awake.

"Why are you here so early?" Katie bit back her frustration that they would clearly now be late and smiled at her mum.

"We have an appointment. Can you get dressed quickly while I feed the dog?" And clean up in here a bit she thought grimly.

Joan stood in her bedroom trying to think what to do next. She knew Katie was there and a bit cross, although she couldn't imagine why. The dog had finally stopped barking. Again, Joan had no idea why. She tried to remember all Katie's instructions; she had put newspaper down to protect the carpet when the dog came in from outside and she had made her own dinner. One of those awful readymade meals Katie had insisted on buying for her. It wasn't very nice and even the dog had turned her nose up. Joan had tried really hard to chew through the cold lumps of vegetables though she hadn't attempted the meat. That was yesterday. Now what was it she was supposed to do today? She could hear Katie telling her to hurry but what was she meant to do?

"Oh Mum you haven't even started to dress!" Katie had come up the stairs to investigate. She paused, fixed a smile on her face and ushered her mother into the bathroom. "You brush your teeth," she said handing her mother her toothbrush, "I'll find you something to wear."

Joan's bedroom was chaotic, clothes spilled out of the wardrobe, while piles of unwashed underwear and socks sat on the floor. It was only a few days since Katie had been upstairs and she had to fight back tears as she realised just how bad her mother had become. She rummaged in the wardrobe until she found something clean and suitable, pulled fresh underwear from the drawer and called to Joan.

"I'll just go downstairs a minute. Can you pop these clothes on and we will be good to go."

Obediently Joan started to remove her night clothes. Before she left Katie spotted the stains down the front of her nightie. She wondered when her mother had last done any washing. Despite her earlier resolve she hadn't had a chance to do a thorough search for dirty clothes in the last few weeks. However, Joan had been adamant she had put everything in her laundry basket or washed it herself and it was easier to believe her.

All Katie really had time to do was to clear the dog's mess and scrape the wasted food into the bin. She realised with alarm that the "easy cook" ready meal had not been cooked at all. She stacked dishes in the dishwasher and turned it on. Joan was finally coming down the stairs, the rest would have to wait.

The journey to the memory clinic was relatively painless. Katie left the radio on with nice, soothing, classical music. It helped numb her senses as Joan carried on her usual habit of pointing out people and places she had never seen and remarking on them as though they were constants in her life. It no longer alarmed Katie that every pub had been lunched in, every river walked by and every man with a hat was always wearing that hat, but it irritated her and made the awful twist of loss much more apparent. Her mother was gone; who was this woman? Hopefully today there would be some answers.

"So, when did you last do any washing Mum?" she asked. "Do you need a new set of instructions?" Katie had painstakingly written careful instructions for each of Joan's appliances and stuck them on the fronts a while ago now after an internet site had suggested it.

"I rinse my underwear out in the basin every night," said Joan." There's no need to put a machine on just for me."

"But what about your clothes?"

"Things don't get that dirty; I don't really do very much and I've plenty to wear." Katie grimaced to herself. Clearly, her mother's washing was going to have to be permanently added to her family's.

They pulled into the hospital car park 10 minutes after the appointment was due to start. Katie grabbed her handbag and ran to buy a pay and display ticket. Opening her purse, she discovered she had no change. Joan was still sitting in the car. She raced back; "Mum do you have any change?"

"I'll look dear." It took an age for Joan to rummage in her handbag and find her purse. Then even longer to open it and discover a mass of small coins.

"How much do you want dear?"

"I'm not sure, let me take your purse to the machine Mum." Katie let the impatience win as she grabbed the purse and ran back to the machine. Slowly the machine swallowed a multitude of 10 and 5 pence pieces until the required £2.00 had been reached. She turned back to the car. Joan was gone!

She scanned the car park and spotted her walking in the wrong direction.

"Mum!" she yelled as she dashed back to the car, stuck the ticket on the windscreen and slammed the door.

"Mum come back you are going the wrong way!" Joan turned bewildered and started to walk towards Katie.

"No need to be cross dear, we always go that way so why should today be different?" Katie resisted the urge to yell that Joan had never to her knowledge set foot in the place before and instead linked her arm through her mother's.

"We are going this way today Mum and we are a little late so let's get going, shall we?" By the time they reached the waiting room, another 7 minutes late, Katie was terrified they would be turned away. She sat her mother down and went to the reception desk. They had to speak through a telephone, so she lifted the receiver.

"Joan Jessup, for the memory clinic, sorry we are a bit late, I had a sick child to see to and Mum forgot we were coming..." she babbled.

"You are here now and clinic is running a bit late so you should be OK," smiled the receptionist. "Take a seat, there's coffee in the vending machine if you have any change." Katie smiled weakly, the thought of sifting Joan's small change again dispelling her longing for a strong black and sank gratefully into the chair. Joan sat meekly next to her. Once more Katie was struck by her mother's changed appearance. The lost air and constant state of bewilderment coupled with inexplicable weight gain. How had it got this bad?

A few moments later the doctor called them through. She had the biggest smile of anyone Katie had ever seen.

"Hello, you must be Joan," she said, ignoring Katie, "Please sit down." Joan sat. Katie stood awkwardly, not knowing quite what to do.

"How are you?" said the doctor.

"I'm fine." said Joan.

"Good." said the doctor. "Do you mind if I take your temperature and check your pulse?"

"Of course not doctor," said Joan. Katie found a chair the other side of the room and sat down and watched while the doctor noted Joan's results.

"That's all just fine," said the doctor.

"Good," said Joan.

"So can you tell me how you are feeling today?"

"Quite well thank you."

"Good. I wonder do you feel sad at all?"

"Well yes a bit."

"Can you describe the feeling?"

"Um well yes, I feel useless."

"Why do you feel useless?"

"Because I am so old and I can't remember how to do things and Katie gets cross." The words tumbled out of Joan. Katie froze as she listened.

"I wake up and I don't know who I am or where I am. I try to remember what day it is as I can only phone Katie on the right days, but if I don't know what day it is how do I know if I can phone? I put the telly on to find out, although they never seem to say the day anymore. If I go to the shop and buy a paper then I know, but sometimes I don't want to walk all that way. Sometimes I phone anyway and I get it wrong." Two tears rolled down Joan's face.

"Why is it wrong to phone for help sometimes?"

"Because Katie goes to work on some days and she can't answer her phone then, so I leave a message. "

"Well, that's OK then, isn't it?" said the smiling doctor. Katie swallowed the urge to mutter, not when you get back to 20 missed calls and think the sky is falling in.

"What do you do once you are up?"

"I have my breakfast and take the dog for a walk."

"You have a dog!"

"Yes, she's lovely. Her name is Trixie."

"Where do you take your dog."

"I used to go for long walks. Now I just go to the copse at the end of the road."

"Why?" asked the doctor. Joan just looked down.

"Did you get lost?" asked the doctor gently. Joan nodded.

"How did you feel when you were lost?"

"I thought I might just lie down in a ditch and wait to die."

"Didn't you think to ask for help?"

"There was no one there. I was in the woods. I used to love the woods when no-one was there."

"You know it would take an awfully long time to die," said the doctor. Her smile briefly replaced by a stern expression, "You would have just got cold and uncomfortable. You really don't want to do that."

"Trixie helped!" Joan said brightening. "She knew the way." Katie knew that couldn't be true. Trixie was not that type of dog. She felt sick at the thought of her mum wandering around lost.

"Do you cook for yourself?"

"Sometimes. Lately Katie gets me these horrid ready meals. I don't like them." Katie again resisted the urge to intervene.

"What do you like."

"I do scrambled eggs!"

Katie shook her head gently, hoping the doctor would realise this wasn't true. Her mother hadn't made herself a meal in months.

"Anything else?"

"Well, there's only me so I only need something simple. I like a bit of ice cream too. At my age you can have a few treats."

"Do you catch the bus? To go shopping?"

"Katie takes me!"

"That's nice. What if she were busy? Would you go on the bus?"

"I don't like buses."

"What else do you enjoy?" Joan looked out of the window.

"Flowers," she said unexpectedly. "I like flowers."

"How lovely. Do you have a garden?"

"Yes."

"Do you enjoy gardening?"

Katie thought of the tangled mess of weeds and overgrown grass that passed for her mother's once pristine garden and winced as Joan replied,

"Oh yes very much."

"That's nice. Do you have any help in the garden?"

"Sometimes Katy helps me." Katie shook her head more vigorously this time. The garden had always been beyond her.

"My grandchildren like to play in it."

"You have grandchildren! That's wonderful. How many?"

"Three! Molly and Lucy are the girls. And …and… there's a boy too. He's the oldest you know."

"That's very nice."

"Do you look after your house by yourself?"

"Well yes but it doesn't really get dirty as there's only me."

"OK."

"Do you mind if I do a little test with you?"

"Like in school?" The ever-smiling doctor smiled even wider.

"Did you like school?"

"Oh yes, I was very good at maths!"

"Well, we will have to ask you some maths questions then!" smiled the Cheshire cat.

"That would be lovely."

"But can we start with some other ones?"

"Fire away doctor I'm ready." Sitting across the room Katie marvelled at how skilfully the doctor had won Joan over. She almost jumped when the doctor turned to her.

"Before we start Katie, I assume you are Katie? Could you fill out this form for me?" She handed Katie a sheet of paper then turned immediately back to Joan.

"Right let's make a start!"

Katie looked at the form and then scrabbled in her bag for her glasses. She had left them at home in the rush to get out. The words were too small she couldn't read them.

"I, I seem to have forgotten my glasses, I'm sorry, I had a sick child and I was rushed…"

"You can borrow mine, I don't need them," said Joan airily. Meekly Katie waited while Joan found her glasses and handed them over.

"All set?" asked Joan.

"Yes," whispered Kate.

"Good, I have a test to do you know."

The first few questions seemed standard and Katie was not surprised when her mother didn't know the name of the road the hospital was in. However, that she did not know that she was in the community hospital did shake her. The date obviously was an impossible question, although Katie had expected her to know the season at least. When her mum stated airily that it was 1984, she felt her stomach tighten. Not even the right century!

The questions changed then. Mum had to draw shapes and identify objects. She watched her mother confidently start at 92 and take away in 7s right down to zero. Yet she couldn't draw a cube successfully and worst of all could not recognise the picture of a rhino.

"Not a Hippo but..." prompted the smiley doctor to no avail. Kate felt tears forming behind her eyelids. She blinked them back.

"I'm going to tell you three words now," said the doctor, "then I will time three minutes before asking you to repeat them back to me. The three words are yellow, poppy and velvet."

Joan screwed up her face as though forcing her mind to absorb three such random words. Then unfairly as it seemed to Katie, the doctor distracted her with more drawing till her phone beeped the time was up.

The doctor beamed encouragingly at Joan, "Can you remember the three words?"

Katie felt her hands clench into fists as she willed her mother to know just one of them as Joan shook her head.

"A colour?" suggested the doctor.

Joan's face lit up; "Was it yellow?"

"Yes, yes!" said the doctor, "a flower next, it can be a girl's name too." Joan scrunched up her face,

"Marigold?"

"And a material." Joan shook her head sadly.

"it's quite soft," hinted the doctor.

"Cotton!"

Katie's questionnaire had been full of practical questions about her mother's abilities. She had had to pass the glasses back and forth to Joan so she could do her drawing questions. However, she had managed, she felt, to give a clear picture of her mother's needs. When at last the test was over, she glanced at the clock. They had been there a full hour. She braced herself for the diagnosis and then of course, the solution.

The doctor smiled and looked at Joan. She reached out gently and held both of her hands.

"Well Joan, I think you have done really well today."

"Did I pass my test?" asked Joan brightly.

"You did just fine," smiled the doctor.

"Oh good! See Katie love, your mum still has her marbles!" Katie winced but managed a small smile.

"The thing is," said the doctor, "while you can indeed still do many things, you do seem to have some problems with your memory. I think you know what that means don't you?" Joan looked down and Katie blinked furiously.

"I think you have dementia, probably of the Alzheimer's type. It is still in the relatively early stages so there is still a lot to look forward to. Much that you can still do with perhaps a little extra help here and there. I think also you are a little depressed. I am going to prescribe you some medication. Two types. Are you OK?" smiled the doctor.

"Oh yes doctor, I'm fine."

"The first is an anti-depressant which will lift your mood a little. The second is to help with the dementia. It isn't a cure. In a third of our patients we see some improvement, in a third it slows things down a little and in the last third it has no effect at all. We don't know which group you will be in until we try it." The doctor got up and reached down a large file from the shelf. She handed it to Katie.

"This gives you a great deal of advice on living with dementia. I would suggest you look at the legal aspects first, as there is a limited window for LPA now if you don't have it in place. There are lots of practical tips in there. You can get all kinds of devices to help your mother cope with her day-to-day routine. I would especially advise a clock that displays dates as well as time. Put one in her bedroom and one in the room she spends most time in. Instructions how to make a cup of tea stuck on the wall by the kettle would help, although I would consider turning off her oven and hob at the mains permanently to avoid accidents. You can get healthy, nutritious meals delivered daily; there's a leaflet in your file. I must say you will probably need to look at care options very soon if she is to continue to live alone. As you are her main support you could qualify to attend a free carer's course. It's on Friday afternoons or Monday evenings, although there is a waiting list. There is also a cognitive therapy session which is the most helpful thing we can offer for patients as it usually shows a memory improvement. There is a waiting list for that too. I will put your mother on it."

She turned to Joan then and beamed her biggest smile yet, "Finally we run a lot of research trials. You can choose which ones you decide to do, but can I add you to the list to be approached? Some of them are quite fun. There's singing or exercise classes, all to help your brain. We monitor what effects they have to help us plan for the future."

"I like singing!" said Joan brightly.

"Great! So shall I add you to the list?"

"Yes please!"

"Now we have run over time a bit and you were late, so I do need to move on to my next patient. We will see how you get on and review in six months I think. Have a good look at the file Katie and good luck!"

With that, still beaming broadly, she ushered them from the office. Katie bit back a thousand questions, took her mother's arm and walked her back to the car.

"What a lovely doctor!" said Joan. "Do I have to come back again? Did I pass my test?"

Katie looked at her mother's bright, nervous smile and wrapped her arms around her as she would have Lucy, whispering softly, "Everything's fine Mum, don't worry about anything. I'll take care of it all. Let's go home."

Chapter 22

Afterwards

May 2019

Lucy lay in bed staring at the twinkly stars her mother had stuck on her ceiling. They glowed in the dark which she found quite comforting. Mummy had also painted a big sun and moon on the walls and a pretty scene of flowers and trees with three little rabbits. Sometimes she thought she was getting too old for it, although mostly she just enjoyed looking at it and knowing her mummy did that for her.

Today Mummy wasn't there. Her tummy hurt and she didn't want to swallow even the water her daddy kept giving her as she felt sick every time. Mummy had been cross that she was ill and left her. Daddy was cross he couldn't go to work, so he was downstairs on his computer. He kept coming in and making her drink. He never helped her get up and go to the toilet and she had wet the bed. She lay there wondering what she had done to make everyone so angry. She didn't dare tell her daddy about the bed. He wouldn't like that at all. Instead, she lay there, wet, cold and miserable, hoping Mummy would come home soon.

Joan sat in the car staring out of the window. She knew she had seen a doctor who had told her she was ill, although she couldn't remember what she had? Was she going to die? She had done a test too, she wondered what that was for. Was she going back to school? She laughed out loud at the thought and Katie glanced at her quizzically. Joan didn't tell her the joke; Katie might not understand. Instead, she focussed on looking for familiar landmarks. There was that man in that hat again. He was always walking along this street. So was the man in his string vest! He must be cold. And the lady with the dog. The dog looked like Trixie. Trixie! She had been left a long time! Did she need feeding? Had she walked her? She started to breathe rapidly as she struggled to remember.

"Katie! I need to get back for Trixie!"

By the time they reached Joan's house Joan appeared to have completely forgotten where they had been. Katie sent her off for a walk with Trixie and decided to wait to be sure she came back. She spent the time stuffing dirty clothes into a bin bag to take home with her and mopping the kitchen floor. The dishwasher had run while they were out, so she carefully put everything away. She was just about to attack the bathroom when Joan reappeared.

"Katie love what a nice surprise! I'll put the kettle on!"

Katie was by now desperate to get back to check on Lucy. It was almost lunchtime. First, she needed to make sure her mother ate. Jack was there after all. Surely, he could cope for one day. She opened the fridge. A pungent smell of who knew what assailed her.

"I know Mum let's pop to that little café down the road. Let's treat ourselves." She made a mental note that her next day's job was to purge the fridge and hurried Joan back out of the door.

Service in the café was slow and her mother struggled to choose from the menu. Once she had her food she tucked in and ate every scrap of her fish and chips. She had settled on that, "as it's Friday you know". It wasn't of course. Katie had forced down a salad sandwich.

"Can we have dessert?" asked Joan.

"I don't really have time Mum sorry…" Joan looked crestfallen like a little child denied a pudding. It had been a tough day. Maybe she needed a treat to lift her spirits.

"OK Mum but we need to take it with us." They left the café with Joan licking happily at an ice cream cornet.

It was 2.30 when Katie finally turned the key in her own home. She wanted to rush upstairs to Lucy, but Jack stood in her way, glowering.

"Well?"

"Mum has dementia."

"Tell me something I don't know! Why did it take so long? I've been stuck here all day and have had to cancel numerous meetings. The boss is not happy. I absolutely must make my 3.00pm meeting. I will probably be very late home. "

"And how's your daughter?"

"In bed as you instructed. I've made sure she kept drinking. Now get out of my way I need to go!" Katie watched his retreating back for a second before running up the stairs.

Lucy looked tiny and frail tucked right up under her duvet. Her eyes were wide with what looked like fear. Puzzled Katie rushed to her side and scooped her up in her arms.

"I'm so sorry sweetheart I had to take Grandma to the hospital. How are you feeling?"

Lucy's big eyes filled with tears.

"Don't leave me with Daddy again. He's mean."

"I won't I promise."

"Good! Is Grandma OK? Was she very ill?"

"She is fine now, but the doctor had to do some tests…." Katie stopped; she could feel something wet.

"Did you spill your drink sweetheart." Lucy bit her lip and slowly shook her head.

"What happened; why is your bed so wet?" Big tears trickled down Lucy's face,

"I couldn't help it. I felt too ill to walk to the toilet by myself."

Katie ran Lucy a warm bath full of bubbles and after washing her down, gently wrapped her in a warm towel. She had rung Molly's best friend's mum who had kindly agreed to bring Molly home as Lucy was too ill to go out to collect her. She stripped Lucy's bed, but the mattress was wet, so she tucked her up in her own big double bed. By this time Lucy was smiling and felt she could manage a little bit of toast. After watching her eat it, Katie read her a story before tucking her down for a nap.

"I'll be back up as soon as I have loaded the washing machine," she said. She handed Lucy a little silver bell that had been her mother's. "While I'm gone if you need me, you ring this bell and I will come running."

Lucy lay in her mother's big bed. She was glad Mummy was being kind now. But Grandma must be terribly ill if Mummy had had to leave her so long. She wouldn't ask about it, she didn't want to make Mummy sad. She closed her eyes and at last slipped off to sleep.

Katie loaded the washing machine with Lucy's bedding first. Her mother's clothes would go on next. Molly was home and doing her homework. Matt should be arriving any minute and she needed to think of what to make for dinner. And what to tell them about their grandma. And Jack…she needed to think about Jack…but not now, not today.

The big, thick file sat on the kitchen table unopened. Maybe it had some answers inside it. Maybe tomorrow she would read it. Then again, she was working tomorrow. So maybe not. She reached for her phone. The school policy was that you had to have adequate childcare even for a sick child. She had none. She knew the Deputy Head wouldn't be happy, but she couldn't leave Lucy again. Biting back the urge to throw the phone at the wall and sit on the floor and sob she started to scroll through the numbers for the Deputy's home one. Instead, she found her counterpart. The lady she job shared with. Just maybe she would swap days.

Joan was settled in her comfortable chair, Trixie on her lap and the TV on. She had been out for a lovely meal with Katie. They'd been for a drive too, never mind that she couldn't remember where. Though they had seen that man again. The one with the string vest. He must be so cold! She chuckled to herself as she drifted off to sleep.

Chapter 23

Jack

May 2019

It took Katie a few days before she could tackle Jack. Her job share hadn't been able to cover for her and had told her to simply tell school she was sick, not her daughter. Any vomiting bug meant 48 hours off work so no one would query it. Katie hated lying yet knew she had to be with Lucy. As it turned out Lucy was feeling much better and they spent a lovely day playing board games, doing puzzles and curling up on the sofa to watch 'Frozen', "just once more Mummy!" She rang her mother a few times and found that Joan had totally forgotten her 'test' and instead happily chatted about mysterious things 'Katy' had told her.

On Saturday she had to catch up with her chores and risked a quick dash to her mother's while Lucy was watching TV with Molly. Jack was around and she carefully left the girls with tissues, tumblers of water and light snacks. She only stayed long enough to ensure Joan had a good lunch and that Trixie had been fed and let outside.

No matter what she was doing Jack's attitude was festering in her brain. She could barely speak to him when they passed and she knew he was aware of her unhappiness. Equally after years of living with him she knew he would never confront a problem first. She would need to raise it and she had to be feeling calm and confident before she did. That meant she needed to be sure her little girl was fully recovered, her house was under control and her mother was not going to interrupt.

On Sunday morning she carefully folded the last of the washing and put it away. Lucy and Molly seemed to be settled playing with Lucy's dolls house. Matt was at football practice. Purposely she switched off her phone and went to find Jack.

"We need to talk."

"What about?"

"You, us, Lucy, my mother."

"That's quite an agenda. Are you sure that covers it all?"

"Don't be sarcastic Jack. How could you leave Lucy to wet herself like that."

"Me leave her! You left her!"

"You were looking after her and you left her unable to get to the toilet."

"How was I supposed to know she would need that kind of help. Your instructions said make sure she drinks lots and let her sleep. They didn't say anything about toilets."

"Oh Jack I would have thought that was obvious. You drink, you need the toilet." Katie could feel the sarcasm in her own voice now. She had wanted to be calm, but Jack was being ridiculous.

There was a long pause. Jack's face clouded and then he turned and walked away. At the door he stopped and looked back over his shoulder, "Actually it isn't obvious to me. Nothing about Lucy or any of your children is obvious to me. You never let me share them."

"Stop! What did you say? What on earth do you mean? My children."

But Jack was gone.

Later as they lay side by side, but a thousand miles apart, Katie softly whispered:

"Jack, what did you mean?" Jack turned over and closed his eyes.

"Jack, I mean it I need to know what you meant." When he still didn't answer she sat up and turned on her bedside lamp.

"I'm not going to let you sleep until you tell me. I have never excluded you from our children's lives. You were always at work, so I just got on with it. But now I work too and it is only fair you help with the children a bit more. For goodness sake it was only one day!" Slowly Jack pulled himself upright and stared at Katie.

"Just like that is it. You decide to change the rules. You made them; I think it only fair you stick to them. Now I have a big presentation tomorrow so I am either going to go to sleep now, here, or I will go and sleep on the couch, but I will not discuss this tonight."

"When then?"

"Make an appointment with my secretary." Grabbing his pillow and pulling a blanket from the spare linen box Jack left the room.

For the rest of the week Jack and Katie stumbled around each other barely speaking. The fact that the children seemed oblivious bothered Katie almost as much as the obvious tension. When had their lives come to this? Then Friday morning, as he left for work Jack paused and looked at Katie.

"Book a sitter for tonight. We'll go out to eat. We need to talk."

Katie had no idea if the agency they occasionally used would be able to find someone in time, so she made ringing them her first priority, once she had dropped the children off. Then in her break time instead of checking up on her mother, she cancelled Molly's planned play date, moving it to the next week. She couldn't expect a sitter to manage an extra child and knew Molly's friend's mother would expect her to be there if she had a child over. All the time she cursed Jack for dumping this on her and for his assumption that she could just drop everything. She knew Molly wouldn't make a fuss even though it wasn't really fair on her. All through the day as she taught, marked and drove she rehearsed over and over what she wanted to say to him. How unfair he was being, how tough her life was, how much he needed to help her more. She was definitely going to set him straight! However, every time the question of what happened after she told him crept into her head, she swatted it firmly away.

The sitter was a new one so had to be shown where everything was. Matt stomped upstairs saying he didn't need a babysitter and Molly had uncharacteristically cried when told her friend wasn't coming. Only Lucy had seemed excited to have a new adult to lavish attention on her and was busily showing "Suzie" all her dolls when Katie and Jack left. He had booked a restaurant and they drove in silence. It wasn't until the waiter had taken their order that Jack turned to Katie and really spoke.

"You need to turn your phone off, so we won't be disturbed. Don't panic I gave the sitter mine for emergencies. I won't have your mother's endless needs interrupting this."

Katie bristled at the tone as she switched her phone to vibrate and slipped it onto her lap. She wasn't going to be entirely cut off from her children. The agency always used her number. Besides experience had taught her that her mother's real emergencies only happened when Katie was out of reach. She tried to smile at Jack, hoping to soften the mood after all. She was tired, scared and despite her earlier bravado was not ready for a showdown.

However, Jack had set his agenda and he was going to roll with it.

"There are three things you need to hear me say before you sit in judgement of me anymore. I appreciate you don't see my point of view at all and perhaps this conversation should have happened before you started your job, although if you recall you just went ahead and applied without any kind of discussion."

"That's not true! I told you I was looking for a part time job!"

"Looking yes but not applying. You never even told me you had an interview."

Katie coloured realising Jack was right. She had been turned down so many times she had decided not to tell Jack about the last interview. She hadn't wanted to have to explain her disappointment yet again.

"I thought you would be pleased for me."

"Why?"

"Because it was important to me!"

"And that is my second point. You make a lot of assumptions about an order of importance. I don't figure anywhere on that list at all."

"Whoa! What on earth does that mean!"

"It means my third point. You changed everything for yourself, which inevitably affected me and yet you assumed it would all be fine as it was important to you. Not once did you consider my needs."

"Aren't you old enough to deal with those yourself!"

Jack laughed, a hollow, hurt laugh, "Once upon a time fulfilling my needs was the most important thing in your world."

"That was before three children and…"

"Quite."

"Jack, I don't get it. What exactly are you trying to say?"

"Are you ready to listen and not interrupt? Or judge?" Clenching her fists to stop herself from reacting, Katie forced a half smile and nodded.

"When we were first married, we fell into a kind of routine. You cooked, I washed up and so on. We spent Saturdays on chores, I mostly did the garden, you mostly did the house. Then Matt was born and everything shifted. You said you were going to give up work and be a full-time mum. We didn't talk about it properly, you just decided. I could see how happy you were, so I didn't argue. As the bills still needed paying, I had to take on more clients, work longer hours."

"That's not strictly true Jack; we did talk about it and you agreed it was best."

"You said you wouldn't interrupt. But as you have, like I said, I didn't argue. You didn't acknowledge my truth. That it made my life more difficult. I tried very hard not to mind. I loved coming home to my little family. However, more and more Matt would be asleep when I got in. I wanted to give him a cuddle and you would tell me not to disturb him as you had only just got him down. I wanted to ask why you did that before I got in, but you looked so worn out from caring for him that I didn't like to. Then when I was there at weekends you made me feel so useless. I couldn't feed him as you were doing that yourself and after my one ill-fated attempt at a nappy change you never let me try again. You just whisked him away to deal with his needs. And so it went on. You went on playdates, to parks and soft play centres. You watched him crawl, walk, speak, run. I was at work and missed it all. I grew to love hearing your tales of your life together and as you made me nice dinners and kept the house in good order it became the new normal. Then Molly came along and nothing much changed except I had to work even harder and you were even more tired. Still, you kept everything spinning and when I was exhausted after a long day at the office, I could only marvel at my amazing wife and my two beautiful children. I didn't want a third. I thought we were fine as we were. I don't even know how we managed to conceive her as neither of us had any energy anymore. You insisted you could manage and after the initial chaos, slowly, as the others set off to school you seemed to draw us all back into some kind of equilibrium. It was all fine again. Peaceful even. Then just as Matt was about to enter adolescence with all its challenges and Lucy was only just starting out at school you decide you need to unbalance life all over again. If you want the mortgage on the bigger house we had to have as you had to have another baby, to get paid, I can't work any less. Yet suddenly after years of exclusion you want me to be daddy day care whenever the mood takes you. You act like I'm letting you down by not doing my part in something you never let me join in the first place." He paused for breath,

"Katie, you look like a goldfish!"

Katie started to laugh. A mad hysterical laugh. She laughed so hard she started to choke and cough. Jack looked around anxiously as people were starting to stare.

"Katie! Stop!" he hissed, but still she laughed and coughed. Tears spurted from her reddening eyes until eventually she put her head into her napkin to try to stem the coughing. Finally spent and exhausted she looked up at her bewildered husband.

"I have never felt like we were a line in 'Gone with the Wind' before but 'it seems we have been at cross purposes my dear,' is all I can think of to say. I'm sorry, I'm not hungry. I'd like to leave."

The sitter had been surprised to see them home so early, although she had been happy to leave once she had been paid for the full evening. Jack had left a large tip in the restaurant with a hasty apology that his wife didn't feel well and they had driven home in painful silence. Once there Katie had gone straight to bed. She didn't get up in the morning. She stayed in bed half the day, alternately sleeping an exhausted but fitful sleep and staring at the ceiling unable to frame her thoughts. Jack had stayed on the couch and she assumed the children were OK as she occasionally heard them pass her door. She had forgotten her phone was off so assumed her mother was coping without her for once. She felt oddly detached from her surroundings, like she was floating away untethered by anything she recognised. It was strangely pleasant and horribly wrong.

"Mummy."

Katie jerked out of her reverie as a little face appeared by her bed.

"Yes Lucy."

"Do you need me to take you to the toilet?"

"No sweetheart I can do that by myself."

"OK-, only Daddy said you were poorly like I was, so I thought I should check." Katie stared at her smallest child and then pulled her into a warm embrace.

"I'm fine sweetheart, not poorly just tired. I'll get up now and maybe you and I can play together today. Would you like that?" Lucy looked confused.

"Don't you have lots to do like always on a Saturday?"

"No not today. Today I am just going to play. Just let me get dressed, OK?" Lucy grinned and skipped off to find some toys. She wasn't quite sure what had happened but clearly it was a Good Thing!

Chapter 24

Jack Part II

May 2019

Katie was loading the dishwasher after a tense, silent Sunday evening meal when Jack tentatively approached her. She looked into his tired eyes and felt nothing but sorrow. Throughout the weekend, a creeping realisation that her relationship with him was the most important issue in her life, had softened her attitude. Unexpectedly she had realised that saving her marriage must come first, when until this crisis she hadn't even understood it was in trouble.

"I can't sleep on the couch again tonight. I'm too tired. I have a presentation to new clients tomorrow. Besides the children are starting to worry."

Katie bit back her reactive, 'You noticed' and instead she nodded at him,

"I'll swap."

"That isn't a permanent solution though is it." Katie shook her head.

"Do you want me to move out?" Again, she shook her head.

"That's a relief."

Once more she bit back her instinctive, 'is it?'. As she did, she found herself questioning how long she had been reacting so sharply to everything Jack said. Why was she so angry at him all the time? Was his version of their life even a little bit true? She smiled gently.

"We need to try talking again don't you think? Perhaps with no one's agenda leading the way."

Jack nodded at her suggestion. "When?"

An image of the week ahead tumbled through Katie's mind. She didn't want to go out again after the last disastrous attempt, equally she didn't want the children to hear. Yet with all her many responsibilities she wasn't sure if a moment would present itself unless they planned. Tentatively she offered an idea,

"Is there a lunchtime you could get away for an hour? We could meet in the park opposite where you work? On Tuesday, Wednesday or Thursday?"

"What about your mum? Don't you lunch with her every day you aren't at work?"

"I can leave her with a sandwich or a salad."

Jack nodded, "Wednesday works best for me. No clients in, just lots of paperwork to do. I can take a long lunch and work back if I need to finish up."

Katie smiled, "It's a date."

Jack turned to leave, then hesitated, "It's a big bed. We can share without meeting in the middle you know."

Tears prickled Katie's eyelids. "I know," she paused, then added softly, "I hope we can meet in the middle again soon."

The picnic was a fantastic idea. Outside, with the sunshine on their faces and no distractions, Jack and Katie relaxed and talked more openly than they had in years. Katie marvelled at her lack of perception over the last six months and beyond. She had been so focussed on the fact that she was drowning, she hadn't seen Jack was slipping under the water beside her just as fast. Now they had the chance of building, not quite a lifeboat, but at least a bit of driftwood to hold on to. They focussed mainly on the practical issues, although inwardly Katie felt that if those improved, the emotional difficulties would ease as well. Jack was certainly far less belligerent and much more open to ideas than in the restaurant. It was as if all the bluster had come out then and now, since he had aired his grievances, he could focus on fixing things. She was happy to go along with anything that helped make life bearable again.

By the end of the lunch, they had some plans. Katie was going to use some of her earnings to employ a cleaner for a couple of hours to do her mother's house for her. Jack was going to take over the football run on Saturday mornings, to strengthen his father son relationship with Matt, by showing an interest in his great passion. Katie could then spend some quality time with Lucy and Molly. Instead of always visiting her mother over the weekend, Jack agreed to collect Joan and bring her to their house for a good old-fashioned Sunday roast once a fortnight. Then the next time Jack wanted to visit his parents Katie was going to go too. That made her anxious at the thought of leaving her mother for a whole weekend and so Jack tentatively raised the issue of care.

"You could get some help you know."

"Who from. There's only me. Mum was an only child and so am I."

"I know that, but there are plenty of care companies out there you know."

"I won't put her in a home. She would hate that. And what about her dog?"

"I don't mean a home. I mean a care company that visits. They go in and make sure your mum has what she needs, eats properly and so forth."

"What about the cost."

"Your mum must have some savings. Perhaps now is the time to use them."

"I don't know if she does."

"Did your LPA come through yet?"

"Well yes, it has been registered."

"So now is the time to use it. Go to the bank and find out what she has. "

"I'm not sure Mum will like that."

"Take her with you then. Let her be involved. "

"I'm not sure she would like a stranger in her house either."

"Perhaps not at first. But these people are trained, aren't they? Hopefully they would start to feel like a friend coming in."

"Perhaps. Oh Jack it is all just so awful. Watching her disappear bit by bit. "

Jack paused, his eyes boring into her face.

"Yes, it is horrible watching someone you love slowly vanish."

She reached out and squeezed his hand. "I'm still here Jack. I'm not going anywhere."

Chapter 25

Crash Course

June 2019

The letter looked insignificant when it arrived, so Katie shoved it into the 'junk mail to be dealt with later' pile and hurried on out of the door. Joan had a hair appointment, followed by the dentist, then the optician and Katie wanted to get her through them all on time. She was starting to think it had been crazy to organise them all on one day. Although with her schedule, it had seemed a good plan when she did it. Joan was in dire need of a haircut and Katie didn't know when she had last seen a dentist. The opticians had been Katie's own idea. If her mother needed glasses and didn't have them, it could be making her symptoms worse. They were all in the same parade of shops so in theory it should work just fine. As long as she could get her mother out of the house on time and everyone was running to schedule.

Joan was up. Although she wasn't dressed, she was at least out of bed and eating breakfast. She knew Katie was coming as it was written in big letters on her white board. There were other things on there too, however Joan didn't bother with those. Reading was such hard work these days. She would let Katie deal with whatever else was on there.

Katie felt rushed and flustered but was pleased her mother was up. She took three deep breaths and tried to calm herself before she went in. She was learning to go at her mother's pace and accept she would have to deal with the unexpected every time she visited. She greeted her mother with a big smile and complemented her on being up on time, while letting Trixie out the back door.

"Where are we going?"

"To the hairdressers. It is time you had a treat." Katie thought one thing at a time would be enough.

"Oh how lovely. What shall I wear?"

"Let's go up and find something shall we? Then you can brush your teeth and we can go."

She helped her mother choose a pair of clean trousers and a blouse and left her to put them on. She fed Trixie and changed her water. Then washed up the breakfast bowl and some random plates and dishes in the sink. They needed to leave in the next five minutes.

"Are you ready Mum?"

"What for?"

"To go out."

"Where are we going?"

"To the hairdressers."

"How lovely. What shall I wear?"

This time Katie stayed with her mother and helped her put on her clothes. She squeezed some toothpaste onto her mother's brush, making a mental note that she needed a new one and got them out of the house about five minutes late. Trixie looked so forlorn as they left that Katie decided to pop her in the car with them. She could walk her round the block while Joan was having her hair cut. She had planned to get some marking done but the little dog's need seemed greater.

The hairdresser greeted Joan like a long-lost friend and she was soon happily settled in the chair, chattering away and drinking tea. Katie slipped out the door to rescue Trixie and take her to a little green patch she had spotted on the way in. Joan's appointment should take an hour and they had an extra 30 minutes after that before the dentist. Katie relaxed and enjoyed watching Trixie gamble across the grass. The exercise was good for them both and marking could wait.

With Trixie settled back in the car, Katie swung the door to the hairdressers open with a smile. Joan should be all ready to go. Her smile vanished as she saw Joan still in the chair with her hair pinned up in tight little curlers.

"What's going on," she asked aghast.

"I'm having my hair done," beamed Joan.

"What exactly are you having done Mum?"

"Um I'm not sure, but the lady said it would look nice."

Katie turned to the hairdresser who was busy cutting another client's hair.

"What is my mother having done? She should be finished by now."

"Her hair was very neglected and we thought a perm would give it some body. She chose the style and seemed very happy. I explained the extra time and cost to my client."

Katie swallowed her wish to scream, "She has Alzheimer's!" and instead simply asked. "How long will she be? We have a dentist appointment in 30 minutes."

"She didn't mention that."

"No…she forgets things. Will she be ready?"

"No."

"How late?"

"I need another hour."

Katie sighed. She would have to whiz to the dentist and explain.

The receptionist in the dentists was very understanding as she explained that no, it would not be possible to push the appointment back half an hour as that would affect all the other patients. Katie had known that really before she asked, she had just felt she had to try.

"Will you want to rearrange?"

Katie sighed. She would quite like to rearrange her whole life into one where Alzheimer's didn't figure!

"Yes please."

The receptionist scrolled carefully down her screen.

"Do you have a particular need to see Dr Sharma?"

"No, I'm happy to see anyone."

"Well, we have a new dentist who started this month. Dr Ashwari. She is newly qualified. I would have to move your mother onto her list permanently, then I could get her in this afternoon at 2.00pm."

Katie mentally ran through the idea. The optician's appointment was at 12.30. They could grab a quick bite in the café next door before seeing the dentist. After that she would have to take Joan with her to pick up the girls from school and then drive Joan home with them tired and hungry. The positive side being that all the appointments would have been done. Her marking would have been abandoned and the washing she had loaded this morning wouldn't be transferred to her dryer. Nor would dinner be started on time. However, her mum could have dinner with them, so at least she would have had a good meal. She could zip her home afterwards while the children watched some TV.

"That will work thank you."

"We will see you at 2.00pm then."

"Oh and could you please warn the dentist Mum has Alzheimer's."

"Is that on her records?"

"No, it wouldn't be. She hasn't been here for ages and has only just been diagnosed."

"I can add it, although your mother will be asked to do a medical form when she comes in anyway."

"Ok thanks." Katie couldn't bring herself to explain how her mother didn't accept or understand her diagnosis and would not be able to do any kind of form. Explaining that was just too much effort. She always assumed if people knew they would respond differently to her mother. She was rapidly discovering they didn't. Unless of course it was to take advantage, she thought grimly.

Back at the hairdressers she managed to mark four books while Joan beamed through her blow dry. She had to admit her hair looked so much better for the perm. Finally, it was time to pay. Joan got out her debit card and tapped it on the machine.

"It's more than £30 you will need to put your pin in," said the hairdresser. Joan looked blankly at Katie.

"Do you remember Mum. Four numbers?" Joan shook her head.

Katie reached into her own purse and pulled out her card. Thank goodness she had her own money now so Jack would never know.

"Do you want to book a six week appointment for a trim?"

"Do I Katie?"

"We need to check your schedule Mum," said Katie firmly, as she pulled open the door ignoring the large jar labelled 'tips'. Find another hairdresser more likely she thought, but Joan's happy smiling face was perhaps worth the inconvenience of the day. She really did look thrilled with her transformation.

"Where are we going now dear?"

"To the opticians. It is only two doors down."

"Why? My eyesight is fine."

"Yes of course it is, we just need to check it out."

"Why?"

"Well as you get older sometimes your eyes get worse. You might need help reading."

"I can read just fine!"

"OK Mum let's go in and show the eye doctor just how well you can do. I bet she will be really impressed."

"Do you think so?"

"Oh yes. She will love your beautiful hair too."

Katie ushered her mother through the door, glancing guiltily at Trixie in the car. The poor dog was going to spend far too long in there. At least it wasn't a hot day and she had left the window open a bit. She would have to let her out at some stage. Maybe Molly would give her another walk later to make up for the time in the car. Although how she would squeeze that into their day, she had no idea.

The optician was a totally different experience. She was calm, professional, and seemed to have endless patience. Katie watched astounded as her mother relaxed under her gentle guidance. However, it was obvious to Katie that her mother desperately needed glasses. She failed to read any except the largest letters and then only after screwing up her face and concentrating hard.

At the end of the examination the optician turned to Katie and smiled, "There is another test I would like to do on your mother; it has an additional charge."

Here we go thought Katie, although she only said, "Why?"

"Well from what I can tell your mother has healthy eyes. However, she does have some difficulty with letter recognition. That could be because something is beginning to develop. Or," she glanced at Joan who was looking away, "it could be to do with her condition. The test I want to run will give me a scan of the eye which will help me determine how much is due to eye problems."

"Are you saying if Mum didn't have Alzheimer's her eyes would be better?"

"I don't have that whatever it was you said! I'm perfectly healthy. And my eyes are just fine! Come on Katie I'm hungry."

Joan looked like a petulant child with her bottom lip stuck out and her hands on her hips.

"Your eyes are remarkably good for your age Mrs Jessup and you did really well on my tests. So much so I would really love to have a closer look at your beautiful eyes if I could please. I can show you the scan afterwards. It makes a lovely picture."

"How much?" asked Katie.

"£40," said the optician.

"I can afford that can't I?" said Joan looking anxiously at Katie. Inwardly grimacing, as because it was over the £30 limit she would have to pay, while outwardly smiling reassuringly at her mother, Katie nodded.

Afterwards Katie was glad she had done the test as it showed clearly that all Joan's problems weren't caused by her Alzheimer's and she definitely needed some glasses. However, the worst was yet to come. Never having worn glasses before, Katie had a vague thought that pensioners got theirs for free. The optician explained gently that no that was just the test (which hadn't all been free in the end), glasses had to be paid for. The frames could cost anything from £25 upwards, but the lenses seemed astronomical. Still, if it helped her mother. She mustered her enthusiasm and pointed Joan firmly towards the cheaper end of the racks.

"Come on Mum let's choose you some nice glasses."

"I don't need glasses."

"Now Mum the lady just tested your eyes and said you would see better if you wore them. Come on, let's find some you like." Katie picked up the nearest pair and held them out to Joan, "Try these."

Katie had to admit that pair looked terrible. They tried a couple more as the optician watched and studied Joan's face. By the fifth unsuitable pair Joan was getting agitated. It was then the optician swooped, grabbing a lightweight pair with a thin gold rim from the mid-price range and holding them out to Joan.

"I think these will suit your face. And work with your pretty hair."

"Really?"

"Try them and see."

Obediently Joan put them on and stared at herself in the mirror. Even Katie had to admit they flattered her mum's face and looked infinitely better than any she had suggested.

"Do you like these?" asked Joan.

"They do suit you Mum."

"Then those are the ones I'll have then."

The optician smiled. "You get to know what suits a face when you do this every day. I will price all that up for you with the lenses and then if you are happy, I will order them in. It takes about a week."

"Can't I take them now?" Joan looked crestfallen.

"It's only a week Mum and then you will look wonderful in them. And they will help you so much." Joan nodded and Katie waited to pay the bill. Her hands shook as she put in her pin number. The total was £365! She knew she had the money; she just did not expect to be spending so much on her mother in one day. She supposed she could ask for it back, although quite how that would work out she didn't know. Did her mum even have £300 to spare? Once more she reminded herself that now her power of attorney had come through, she needed to take it to the bank and sort out her mother's finances.

Joan smiled warmly at the optician, thanking her for her time and they returned to the car to let a grateful Trixie out for a bit. Katie managed to grab an outside table at the café, so they sat with Trixie at their feet and ate cheese sandwiches and cake. Joan had insisted on the cake. My treat she had announced and flourished her card at the counter. Kate had smiled to herself at the irony and thanked her mum for her kindness.

"Last stop now Mum. The dentist."

"Really? But my teeth are fine."

Let's hope so thought Katie as she said, "Just a check-up Mum."

This time it was. A bit of age-related wear and tear, a suggestion that Joan should come back for a hygienist appointment for some cleaning and they were done.

Katie clicked her mother's seat belt in place and they set off to get the girls from school. She had remembered too late that Jack would not let the dog in the house and so poor Trixie was going to have to be confined to the garden while they ate. Still hopefully Jack wouldn't notice she was there and Molly could smuggle her out some food. The day had been too long already and she was not capable of withstanding one of Jack's moods.

Much later, after a frantic evening, with Jack's frustration obvious but unspoken, except over the dog where he made his feelings very clear, Katie was about to sort out the long neglected wet washing when she remembered the letter from the morning. Anything to avoid what might well be smelly washing by now, she ripped it open. She had been invited to go on a course for carers. It was for six weeks and covered all areas of caring. It started the next week and Katie had a choice of Monday daytime or evening. It would have to be Monday she cursed, as that was a workday. How on earth would she convince Jack to babysit for six weeks?

"Jack," she started tentatively, desperation making her brave, "I have been invited on a course for carers.

"When."

"Starts next week."

"What day?"

"Mondays, 7pm for six weeks." She thought it best not to mention the daytime option.

"Typical, evenings, what is it about?"

"Well, there's a week on powers of attorney and other financial matters, one on managing day to day care, one on…"

"OK I think you should go."

"Really?"

"Yes really. Honestly Katie you need some help. Look at today. Anyone could have told you dragging your mum from one place to another like that would end in tears. You won't listen to me, so time to bring in the experts. Maybe they can talk some sense into you."

Swallowing the urge to yell, scream or throw something at him, Katie allowed herself a little wry smile of triumph. Somehow, he had just agreed to take care of the children Monday nights for six weeks! And she was going to get some professional help at last. A course in caring. Hopefully a crash course she thought, as he was right about one thing. Today had not been her best day.

Joan pulled on her nightie and struggled into bed. She was so very tired. She couldn't understand why. She had been with Katie. Had they had lunch out? She thought there were glasses involved somehow, although she couldn't find any now so maybe not. It had been good to see the children though. Shame Jack had been so cross about Trixie. She had only been in the garden. Obviously, he didn't like her. How could anyone not like her little dog. Perhaps that was why she was so tired. She must have walked all the way home with Trixie…

Chapter 26

Course Day 1

June 2019

Katie scanned the room to try to spot an empty seat. All the other participants were chatting animatedly and she knew she was late. She had run through the door to the cottage hospital 5 minutes after they were due to start. She felt that wasn't bad going after a day at work, a phone call to her mum and producing dinner for her family. She hadn't had time to join them but had swallowed a few mouthfuls as she ran out of the door. The older two had done their homework and were allowed TV as long as they were good. All Jack had to do was hear Lucy read and tuck her in to bed. If he didn't succeed, she reckoned she would be home not long after 9.00pm so could pick up the pieces then. And eat. Her stomach growled as she searched again for her seat.

"Are you looking for someone?" An officious looking lady came towards her clutching a clip board and pen.

"I'm here for the course."

"You aren't on my list."

Katie bit back her immediate thought of "How do you know you haven't asked who I am," and simply muttered "I was invited."

"Did you book?"

"I was invited."

"Yes, lots of people are invited. If you want to come you have to book. If you don't book your place is offered to the next on the list."

"I didn't know that."

"The reply slip was in the envelope."

Again, Katie wanted to scream "How do you know that! I would have seen it." Then remembering the day she opened the letter, she realised she might not have.

She tried a different tack. Fixing her best, brightest smile on the woman she said, "Well now I'm here I might as well stay."

"Oh no we don't have your details. And our speakers won't have enough handouts. And", Miss Clipboard said triumphantly, "there aren't any more chairs!"

"You can share mine," said an unexpected voice.

Katie spun to see a gentle smiling face, "Handouts that is. I don't think we could both fit on one chair. Although I did spot some in the corridor. Shall I fetch one while you give the lady your details? We can easily squeeze it in next to me."

Miss Clipboard muttered darkly about "procedures and fire numbers," then shrugged and took down Katie's name and address while Katie herself slipped gratefully into the fetched chair.

"Thanks, I'm Katie," she whispered as the speaker was about to start.

"Jackie, glad to help, officious old bat!"

"Alzheimer's is only one form of dementia…" began the speaker, glancing sharply at Katie and her new friend as they stifled their giggles.

To begin with, Katie was vaguely disappointed by the first evening. Lots of information thrown at them from a distant speaker about the forms of dementia and all its possible symptoms. She had read most of that on the internet and couldn't see how anything she was hearing was going to make her life any easier. She did discover that her mum's habit of commentating on everything she saw as though it was familiar was unique to her. At least as far as the speaker knew. Alzheimer's throws up all kinds of possibilities apparently. When you are dealing with the brain there could be any number of variations in effects of the disease. Katie felt absurdly proud that her mum had a unique symptom. For a moment at least, until she realised how crazy that was. Much better not to have what was undoubtedly a hideous disease.

Then as the speaker moved on towards the final devastating few years of a dementia sufferer, she felt tears pricking her eyelids. She knew her mum would eventually forget everything; however, she hadn't thought about her losing the ability to swallow, the loss of mobility, even incontinence. The thought of her bright, happy mum lying in a bed, a totally vacant shell, wearing adult nappies was too much and she felt bile rising in her throat.

"Awful isn't it?" She heard a whisper to her left.

Jackie put a gentle hand on hers. "I'm guessing you are still in the early stages?"

"It's just so unfair."

"And random and cruel and all those words. I have used them all, then in the end, you accept that you can't stop it and just focus on getting through it."

Katie gulped and looked at her new friend.

"Is that what you do?"

"My mum is in a home now. I did all I could to start with, until in the end, it was the safest, fairest option."

"Was your mum OK with that?"

"Not very at first. Now she has simply forgotten she was ever anywhere else."

The speaker shot them a glance.

"Let's grab a coffee and chat after."

Katie thought guiltily of Jack as she nodded.

By the time Katie got home it was almost 10.00pm. Thankfully all the children were asleep and Jack barely glanced up from the TV as she crept through the door. Chatting to Jackie had been the lifeline she needed far more than the course. They had talked about all kinds of other things: family, husbands, home, work, before getting on to their mother's needs. They shared silly stories of their children's antics, mixed with poignant moments when the strain had hurt too much to bear. Jackie had tried for years to keep her mother in her own home, until, as she lived over 100 miles away, the endless trips back and forth had broken her. She had tried care at home and found it was inconsistent and hard to supervise from such a distance. In the end she found a lovely home in the same locality and settled her mother there. She still visited once a fortnight, but it was no longer to clean and cook, just to chat and try to find something of her real mum behind the empty eyes.

While Katie could only sympathise with Jackie's current situation, Jackie had lived Katie's. She knew all about the endless panicked phone calls, the imaginary broken TVs, although in her mother's case it was the radio and the constant need to juggle her family to fit in with her mother's demands. She had listened quietly as Katie poured it all out and then simply stated the obvious,

"You need help!"

Katie had laughed and then swallowed a gulp before blurting, "Where do I get that?"

"Week 2 I believe."

Chapter 27

Money

June 2019

Week 2 was a solicitor explaining the importance of powers of attorney and wills among other things. Katie was tired and as the speaker droned about LPA's and deputies, probate and wills she felt herself drifting. Jackie nudged her awake.

"This stuff is actually really important. If you want to make the decisions for your mum, you need to get the legalities in order."

"I'm the only child, LPA sorted. Not used it yet though," whispered Katie

"Maybe you should have a look at what is there. Care costs."

Those words jerked Katie awake. After last week she had realised her head in the sand day-to-day approach was not going to work. They needed a long-term plan for her mum. And that it seemed did not come cheap. She paid attention for the rest of the session and went home clutching the solicitor's notes. Jack was still awake and agreed to look through them with her. She watched as his brow furrowed and he um'd and argh'd at intervals.

"Right, first things first, you need to see if your mum has a will. It isn't the end of the world if she hasn't, as I don't think anyone exists to make claim on her, but you never know. It will just make life easier…sorry…in the event…you know."

Katie nodded. "I will ask Mum." Jack smiled ruefully, "If she doesn't quite remember, are you aware of a family solicitor or anywhere she keeps documents?"

"Actually yes; she has an old desk in her spare bedroom. She keeps everything important in there."

"That's a good start. The other thing we need to do is go to the bank. Find out what her accounts hold and if she has any savings. Your LPA has been registered, if you show it to them, they will tell you."

"Should I take Mum?"

"No sweetheart. Go alone. It will be easier on you and you don't need to worry her. I can come too if we do it one lunchtime."

"OK."

"And finally, I think we missed something. We did her financial POA but not the health and welfare one. We should get that done as soon as possible. Otherwise, you won't necessarily have the right to choose your mum's future care."

"I'm her daughter! Who else is there?"

"Good question, apparently according to this, being family isn't necessarily enough. The state can overrule unless you have the correct bit of paper. It's OK. I will download and fill it out for you. Then you will need to get your mum to sign it with a witness, like we did the other one."

Katie nodded and putting the papers to one side slipped up to bed. It had been a long day followed by too much information. She was grateful Jackie made it lighter and Jack was being helpful. It was good not to feel so alone.

The trip to the bank didn't quite go as planned. Jack suggested making an appointment, so Katie phoned and asked for a lunchtime one. None were available for at least a month as apparently everyone wanted to pop in at lunchtime. That meant Katie found herself sitting across the desk from a round, smiley lady with a pronounced northern accent on Thursday morning as no one seemed to prioritise their banking then. Katie was glad of the early appointment, although she wished she had Jack with her as she wasn't used to dealing with these kinds of things. She had given in her copy of her power of attorney and the lady had disappeared for a while before coming back with various sheets of paper.

"Right well I have the details of all the accounts your mother holds here in this bank. She may well have other accounts in different institutions, although it seems she runs her day-to-day banking through us.”

“I don’t think she has any others. She has always used your bank, even when I was little.”

“I see. No building society or post office accounts? Lots of older people like to use the post office for savings.”

“I don’t think so.”

“Well maybe she’s the type to hide it under the mattress.” The banker’s attempt at humour scared Katie rather than making her smile.

“Is there a problem?”

“No not as such. Your mother has everything in order.”

“That’s good, isn’t it?”

“Yes.” The banker switched to brusque efficiency. “Her current account shows that her pension goes in every month. She has two, the normal state one and another, presumably from working?” She pointed to the appropriate entries on the papers she had printed.

“Yes, she has been retired about 15 years now, but she always worked. She was a secretary for a law firm.”

“The two together seem to cover her monthly outgoings. Her bills are all a bit random. It seems she pays them in the post office, which as I mentioned is a favourite with the older generation. I would suggest the first thing you do is set up some direct debits. That will spread the costs more efficiently and ensure she doesn’t go overdrawn. Other than those there is nothing much except regular cash withdrawals. A few small cheques. My guess is charity donations. Lots of people out there preying on old folks for their money. Second thing you need to do is hide the cheque book or better still tear it up.”

“Is that fair? I mean surely Mum should still be allowed to give to charity?”

The banker smiled. Up to you lass, but with your mum’s accounts I would think you would want to ensure as much as possible was available for her needs. She will be needing some help I should imagine.”

“Yes, not yet but some time. Surely there is enough for that.”

The banker smiled gently and pointed to the top figure. Katie hadn't noticed it yet; she had been too intent on looking at the in goings and out goings. The total in her mother's account was £29.

"Like I said she keeps within her income, mostly, she went over two months ago, but only by £12.50 and she has an agreed overdraft of £500 so that isn't a problem. There just isn't any spare for her to be giving away or more to the point getting any help in."

"Does…does she have a savings account at all? I mean, she worked all her life. Surely there has to be something more."

"Yes, she has a savings account. Let me find the printout." The banker shuffled the papers while Katie waited anxiously. Her mother had never been extravagant and there had only ever been the two of them, at least since she was very little when her father had died from a sudden heart attack.

"Here, there's the total."

Kate stared. The sum total of her mother's life savings was £2,526.

"I assume she owns her own home?" the banker said gently, seeing the disbelief on Katie's face. "There's no rent or mortgage outgoings."

"Yes, she's lived in our house forever. Well, since I was born. I grew up there. My dad died when I was little. I don't remember him at all."

"Perhaps he left something and it is invested elsewhere?"

"No….I don't think so. Mum had this friend. Auntie Mac I used to call her. Sometimes she would go on about what a shame it was Mum had to work and that Dad hadn't left us better provided for. Mum used to grit her teeth and smile, but it always irked her. She needed her though and she was kind in other ways; she used to pick me up from school and give me tea until Mum got home…sorry here's me rattling on. I hadn't thought about any of that in years. So no, I don't think there's any hidden cash."

"I would still check your mum's drawers though. She might have an account you know nothing about. Anyway, I would encourage you to set up online banking for your mum so you can keep an eye on things. If you want her to keep her card for now that's fine and we can issue one for you too if you want."

"Oh yes please. I do her shopping. That would really help."

"And let's put a £50 limit on your mum's card. That way she can't make any impulsive purchases or be scammed out of large sums."

"Thank you. For all your help."

"No problem love. It can't be easy, but you'll find a way through."

Katie swallowed. Accepting the sympathy of strangers was sometimes the hardest thing to do.

Explaining her mother's financial situation to Jack was not easy. He was horrified to discover how little Joan had put by. She had always appeared financially secure. She had dined out, dressed smartly and travelled quite widely when she was younger. However, it appeared that saving had not been part of her plans. Katie had never felt she went without anything as a child. Appearances were deceptive it seemed, or perhaps it was only since her mother retired that things had got tighter. Jack had been convinced Joan must have an insurance policy somewhere or another savings account. This led to a careful search of Joan's desk drawers. They were very neat and had clearly not been opened for years. Nothing turned up. It was obvious Joan simply lived day to day without any thought for the future and probably had always been that way. Katie expressed as much to Jack.

"I guess when she was left alone with a small child, she just had to cope on a day-to-day basis and over time that became her habit."

"Not a good one though."

"At least she owns her home. That gives her something of real value."

"Yes, that could actually be quite helpful."

"How do you mean?"

"There are ways for the elderly to release some of the value of their home while still living in it. I can get some details from Bob at work. He did it for his parents. They used theirs to fund repairs on their roof, but your mum could use it to fund some care at home."

"I don't want strangers in Mum's house. I don't think she will like it."

"I know sweetheart, but she needs more help than you can give her. At least let's look at getting a cleaner. We talked about it before, but it hasn't happened yet. If we tidy up her expenses and stop all these charitable donations for a start, she can have someone in for two hours a week. That will make a big difference."

"Ok, only if she is happy with that."

"Seriously Katie," Jack pulled his exasperated face, "you are running yourself ragged doing the cleaning here and there as well as all the shopping and cooking. Your mum is going to have to accept some outside help."

"She can be very stubborn you know."

"Like mother like daughter!

Chapter 28

The Cleaner

June 2019

Joan blinked and stared at the stranger on her doorstep. The stranger was smiling and clutching a mop and a bucket full of cleaning items. Behind her on the step was a large Henry hoover, which she pulled along in her wake as she stepped past Joan into the hallway.

"Sorry I'm a bit late, last place was a right mess. But I'll have you sorted in a jiffy; you'll still get your two hours don't you worry. Shall I start upstairs? Don't s'pose you could pop the kettle on, a nice cup of tea really helps in my line of work. Oops hello sweetheart."

The constant stream of words paused as the Mop Lady bent to pat Trixie. Then she set off towards the stairs. Joan stood and watched, unsure what her next move should be. Should she put the kettle on? She decided instead to ring Katie.

As she picked up the phone she looked carefully at the calendar. Was today a 'No phone calls Katie is at work' day? Those were ringed in red with a notice underneath saying 'Katie is at work on red days'. The idea was that Joan crossed off a day each morning, so she knew what day it was. And if she forgot there was a lovely new date and time clock on the mantelpiece to tell her what day it was. She looked carefully at the clock. It said Friday. She looked at the calendar- Fridays were red days. No Katie.

She shook her head. Why was she going to ring Katie?

Trixie was barking and there was an odd noise like a vacuum cleaner upstairs. Joan frowned. What was happening? Someone had been in her house. She was supposed to make tea. Why was the dog barking! Was it Katie upstairs? She put the kettle on.

"Do be quiet Trixie!"

"It's alright love I'm nearly done up here. Your bathroom's sparkling and I've hoovered all through. I'd love that tea now, then maybe I can tackle the kitchen. I'll try and squeeze in hoovering downstairs too, but really you need another hour and then I can get to grips with the dusting, shine up all those knick-knacks of yours. You've got some lovely stuff."

The Voice came down towards Joan trailing equipment in its wake. Joan stared again.

"Ooh how lovely, you have put the kettle on. Shall we have one together? No extra charge for the time, I will do the full two hours regardless, it is just nice to have a bit of a chat with my clients and get to know you a bit. Now where did you get that lovely vase by your bed, beautiful that is. C'mon little dog, bet you'd stop barking if we shared a biscuit!"

Joan poured hot water into two mugs, picked up a packet of biscuits and obediently followed the clattering, heavy laden Voice into her living room.

They sat.

Joan smiled.

"Thank you, this is lovely. Garibaldi my favourite. Not so many people have them these days. My Nan always did. She used to bring them out just for me when I popped in after school. Mind you that was a lot of years ago now back in Cardiff…." The sing song Welsh Voice continued unabated for half an hour.

Joan smiled.

Finally, it stopped. The Voice went back to the kitchen, somehow managing the tea tray as well as all her own clutter.

"I'll wash up these bits now and then do over your kitchen. Why don't you sit there and have a bit of a rest love? I'll be a good 50 minutes in here by the looks of it and then I'll whip the hoover round that room and up the hall. Then I'll be off on my travels to the next stop…"

Joan grabbed Trixie's lead, clipped it on her collar and fled.

"And next thing I knew the door was shutting and she was off without so much as a by your leave. I had no idea what to do. I can't just sit around and wait for clients who wander off. I'd done what you asked, done the extra half hour chat and not told her it was an extra charge, but it seems she didn't like my company and went off on her own…"

"She has dementia…" Katie interjected, although the Voice carried on regardless.

"I can't be hanging around all the time just waiting. I needed to move on to my next client. They like me in and out before they are home and with squeezing in your mum I had to rush to get there as it was, without the extra 20 minutes I waited."

"I'm sorry but…" Katie tried again.

"Next time could you just tell her to stay in or to tell me she is going. As it was, I worked out the door locks when it closes. Bit dodgy that really with an old lady, what if she forgets her keys? Anyway, I decided I could just go as the place was safely locked. But I was that worried about her in case she wasn't allowed out alone and all. You never know with dementia. Are you sure she shouldn't be in a home?"

Katie had had enough.

"Look I am sure you have another job to get to now. Perhaps I can just pay you for the extra 20 minutes and we can call it a day."

"Oh well I did do a bit of dusting while I waited."

"Fine I will transfer a bit extra to cover that."

"You do want me to go back?"

Katie took a deep breath. The Voice, Mrs Nicholls a cleaner she had found online, was starting to sound more worried than indignant.

"I think perhaps not. Mum was clearly upset by having someone she didn't know in the house…"

"I moved everything around to fit you in. I'm sure she will know me next time."

"I really appreciate your efforts and you did a lovely job but sadly Mum won't remember you at all."

"I can remind her who I am."

"Unfortunately, that won't help."

"Like that is it? No second chances."

"I really am sorry it didn't work out, but we did say it was a trial."

After hanging up the phone, Katie initially felt relief. Then she realised she would have to start over in looking for a cleaner. This time she was going to be a bit more thorough and interview them carefully. Until today she hadn't spoken to Mrs Nicholls, simply hired her by email. This was going to be a much harder than she thought. After just one conversation with Mrs Nicholls, she knew she wouldn't suit her mother at all. Still, she felt a pang of remorse for not being more careful. The poor lady was after all just doing her job. She sighed and turned back to her own messy house and picked up a cleaning cloth. She had better begin with the kitchen.

Jackie wiped her eyes from laughing when Katie told her the tale. Coffee after the course was definitely the best bit of Monday evening.

"Don't laugh, poor woman, she was doing her best."

"I know but you have to admit it is funny."

"Well yes, it is. And I totally get why Mum took off. One phone call and I was exhausted. Imagine 30 minutes of that in your house when you have dementia."

"Or even when you don't!"

"To think I paid her extra to do that too!"

"Yes, that is probably the worst part."

"No, the worst part is I don't have anyone to clean Mum's house!"

"You'll find someone."

"I suppose. It's just finding the time to do it while cleaning two houses myself along with everything else."

"Forgive me if I am overstepping here. Obviously, I don't know anything about your personal finances and it is none of my business. It's just you have said you don't need the money from working; that you do it for other reasons. So, when you do find a suitable cleaner why don't you have her do your house too? If you can afford it that is. Not all of it maybe, just the "heavy lifting" bits? That would give you a lot more free time, wouldn't it?"

Katie starred, her mind digesting this idea.

"Jackie you are a genius!"

Chapter 29

Puzzles

June 2019

Lucy gripped Buzz's head tightly in her hand. It was a Saturday and Mummy had said they could do something together. She had come up with a unique idea. She had taken all the puzzles out of the cupboards and stacked them from the front door to the back, going through the living room and dining room to get there. It was amazing how many puzzles the family had amassed over the years. Distant relatives' birthday presents and her mother's firm belief that every child's Christmas stocking should contain something a bit educational, probably had something to do with it. After carefully placing them, Lucy had announced they had to do them all to make a puzzle pathway through the house. They were on their 16th puzzle; one of a set of Toy Story pictures. Easy ones, but Lucy still liked Mummy to help. That was the point, although she couldn't articulate it. When she did puzzles Mummy joined in. If she had chosen Barbies, after a bit she would have been left to get on with it, whatever Mummy had said about playing all morning. However, now the phone had rung and Mummy was deep in conversation. All Lucy could hear was "hmmm, yes, not that one, try again…" She was pretty sure it was Grandma on the phone. It was always Grandma on the phone.

"OK we will be there as soon as we can." Lucy puckered up her brow. They still had 26 puzzles to complete. She knew as she had counted them out; 42 in all. The last ones were the giant piece toddler ones that covered a lot of space. She could do them alone, but no way could she manage the tricky pirate ship and Horrible History ones that had been Matt's. Then there were Molly's map ones. Way too hard, but big enough to fill space and Mummy always liked telling her about the places on the pictures. She could never do those without Mummy. Grandma would just have to wait until they were done. Mummy clearly thought otherwise.

"Sorry Lucy, Grandma is having trouble with her dinner, I need to go and help." Katie was trialling a new company that delivered pre-prepared meals for Joan. They looked nutritious and easy. However, it involved using the microwave and Joan had never really got the hang of that, even before dementia.

"We can go when we have finished the puzzles?"

"We can finish this one."

"But there's 26 more!"

"I know sweetheart, that would take a long time and Grandma is hungry."

"Can't she just have a biscuit?"

"Oh Lucy, she needs her dinner!"

"It isn't dinner time!"

"It is for Grandma. She eats her main meal at lunchtime. Lots of older people do that."

"I can't do the rest without you!"

"I know, we can do them when we get back."

"We? Do you mean I have to go?"

"Of course! You can't stay here alone."

"Mummy you don't understand! I have 26 puzzles to do before Daddy gets back with Matt and makes me pick them all up."

"We will have time. Maybe Molly can help too."

"I don't want her to! It was meant to be just you and me!"

"Well, it will be just you and me in the car. You can choose the CD we put on."

"Why doesn't Molly have to come?"

"Because she is older sweetheart. She and Matt can stay home but you are too little. We have had this conversation before." It was a new idea that Molly would stay. Katie was only allowing it as Jack was due back very soon. No way would he be happy if Lucy was left as well. Nor would she agree to that. Lucy had to come.

"I could stay with her and Molly could help me do the puzzles and then you wouldn't have to!"

"You didn't want Molly to help. You wanted me to."

Lucy stared defiantly at her mother. Her little voice quavered though as she delivered her final blow.

"You don't want to anymore. You would rather be with Grandma. You always stop playing to go to Grandma's, so I want to play with Molly instead."

Katie bit her lip. She looked down at her youngest child. Guilt swirled through her veins and fear followed. She knew she was failing Lucy. Yet she couldn't abandon her mum. Why did it all have to be so hard?

"I do want to play with you Lucy. Very much. And I promise when we get home, we will finish all 26. While you are very important to me and I love you very much, I love Grandma too. And she only has me to help her."

"Why can't Grandma cook her own dinner? That's what grown-ups do."

Katie paused. How much should she tell Lucy; how much would she understand?

"Lucy, do you understand what your memory is?"

"Of course! Its where all the old stuff I used to do is. In my head."

"Well Grandma has an illness that mean lots of her memories have fallen out of her head."

"Like how to cook her dinner?"

"Yes."

"And how to work the TV?"

"Yes."

"Will she forget me?"

Katie tried desperately to remember what the lady on the course had said about telling children how feelings remained even when names were forgotten. How even though dementia patients might not recognise who you are or remember your name, they will still love you. How had she phrased it for a child to understand? Jackie was always telling her to make more notes; she was just so tired on Monday evenings and her mind wandered so. And now was simply not the time for this conversation.

"She won't forget you, Lucy. How could anyone forget you! Now come on let's get your coat."

"If stuff falls out of her memory, how do you know I won't?"

Katie stopped. She crouched down and looked straight at her daughter. Truth is always better she thought. Except to a dementia patient, then it is better to let them believe their own version of reality. That's what the course had taught her. For her daughter a simpler truth was needed.

"She might forget your name sweetheart. One day. Not yet, a long time from now. Even if she does, she will still know who you are. That you are her very special little girl, who she loves very much. That will stay much longer."

"But not always."

"I don't know about always. I do know she is hungry and we need to go and feed her."

"OK."

"Are you sure?"

"Yes. I thought Grandma was just silly making you go and help her all the time. Now I know it's 'cause her head's gone wrong."

Katie wrapped her precious child in her arms, "Yes it has. Although her stomach still works, so let's go and fill it! And later we will do our 26 puzzles."

Lucy carefully placed Buzz's head into the correct space and followed her mother to the door. Something big had just happened and she wasn't sure quite what. It felt good not to be so cross with Mummy anymore. She kind of knew the puzzles would never all get finished, as something else would interrupt. Somehow, that didn't feel quite so important anymore. She was doing something special with Mummy after all. She was helping Grandma remember her.

Chapter 30

The Cavalry

July 2019

By now they were on week 4 of the course. Katie was feeling good. She had sorted her mum's money and after the Mop disaster that still made her chuckle, the new Good Fairy was working out well. That was the name Jackie had given the new cleaner, who slipped quietly in and out of both houses leaving them spic and span.

The best part of it all had been meeting Jackie who gave her sensible advice and was someone to talk to who was further on in the experience of dealing with dementia. The week 3 information had been all about care homes. Katie had no intention of putting her mother in a home and there was clearly no money for care at home. She had listened vaguely to the details of State-run care, dismissing it as she felt her mother wasn't yet at the stage to need that. Nor, after the experience with the cleaners, did she feel Joan would cope with random visits from strangers. Better to carry on doing what she could as Joan was managing for now. Jackie had encouraged her to take more careful note; warning her the future was inevitably worse than the present and at some stage she would need to 'call in the Cavalry,' as she put it. In some shape or another. However, Katie wasn't ready to hear that and was certain Joan wasn't either.

Week 4 began with Jackie and Katie huddling at the back laughing over Lucy's latest antics. Katie was feeling relaxed. It was nearly holiday, meaning she felt less stressed over work. She was now well practiced in making a Monday meal out of the leftovers from the Sunday roast, in order to escape on time to her course. She would be glad when it was over, although she had gathered a great deal of information and even Jack felt it had been useful. All in all, she was feeling rather smug.

"Today we are going to talk about your own mental wellbeing."

Katie shifted slightly in her seat.

"Caring for someone can take over your life and it is very easy to lose yourself in the midst of it. Some of you have a spouse to support you, for some of you your spouse may be less than supportive. Is caring affecting your marriage? What about children or grandchildren? Do you have time for them too or are they feeling the strain of your caring role? Do you work and have trouble fitting in your caring hours around your busy career? Is your job suffering? What about domestic chores? Do you feel overwhelmed with different responsibilities and are you struggling to prioritise? When did you last do something just for you?"

Katie gulped.

"That is a lot of questions to throw at you all at once. What I want you to do now is take a moment to write on your notepads a list of the other responsibilities you have besides your caring role. Then next to it rate yourself, kindly I might add, out of 10 for your level of success in that role. No one else will look at these, it is just to get you thinking."

Katie scribbled furiously. Her marriage, her children, her home, her job. Easy to list them all but how was she doing? She thought hard and added her numbers. None were over 5. Except work. There she felt she was a seven. Her lowest grade was Jack. Just a three. They had been talking more, which was positive, yet deep down she knew she needed to work harder on her marriage. Much harder. Matt worried her with his sullen silence and lack of effort at school, Molly scared her sometimes with her over compliance and Lucy, Lucy just seemed to be drifting away from her. Although the puzzles day had been good, despite the interruption. Then again, when did she last spend a day with Matt? Or Molly? Maybe Lucy was doing best…

"OK I can see some of you found that quite a challenge. And I imagine you have all rated yourselves tougher than you deserve.

Now tell me who has put themselves on the list. Has anyone rated their self-care?"

There was a moment of silence.

Then the smartly dressed lady in the front row spoke out.

"I didn't think I was responsible for me?"

"Well if you aren't who is?"

"My husband!"

Everyone laughed and her husband who was sitting next to her, as always, patted her hand and smiled.

"And I am responsible for him."

"That's lovely."

"We don't have any children. It's just us and Mum. We take care of each other and together we care for her."

Katie's envy for the patted hand disappeared in a wave of sadness for anyone who had no children. Gratitude for hers swamped her and she found herself swallowing tears.

"You clearly have a lovely set up. Not everyone in this room has that, I imagine," here the speaker seemed to hone in on Kate, "there are some of you who are juggling far too much responsibility and feel there is simply no room on your list for yourself. Do any of your lives look like this?"

The speaker displayed a picture of an upside-down triangle. At the bottom was the word "me". Above it, in increasing sizes and various thicknesses were words like washing, cleaning, ironing, walking the dog, playing with the children, homework, cooking, shopping, time with spouse and so on.

"Do you feel like sometimes you are holding up the world?"

"Yes," it came out as a squeak.

The speaker turned to Katie.

"It's a bit heavy isn't it." The speaker's eyes softened as she focussed on Katie. For a moment the room faded and all Katie saw was her compassion.

"Yes."

"So, let's look at lightening your load. All of our loads. Or at least how to make it all more bearable."

The rest of the evening was spent going through the importance of taking time out for yourself, how it lifted your spirits to spend half an hour doing something you enjoyed. The outdoors was highlighted, exercise classes, deep baths and soft candles, music, laughter and having fun however you chose. All helped ease the burdens and make you a better carer, suggested the speaker. Katie listened with the one word 'When!' screaming in her ears.

"Finally, I would like you to go back to your notepads and write down the one thing you would like to do more of to help you cope better this week. Then I want you to go home and do it!"

Katie wrote:

Sleep.

Katie and Jackie were heading for the door when the speaker softly called out, "It's Katie isn't it?"

Katie turned and nodded.

"Do you have a quick moment?"

"Um, yes I suppose so." said Katie.

"I have been watching you through the weeks and I have noticed your burden seems particularly heavy. It can't be easy juggling children, a career and your mother. It is your mother you care for, isn't it?"

"Yes."

"Please don't take this the wrong way, but as part of our caring services we offer a few therapy sessions to carers. No don't look alarmed. It is just a chance to unburden yourself a little and talk through ways to help you. There's no judgement," she added softly, "just support."

Katie looked into her gentle brown eyes. She felt she could easily pour all her fear and doubt into those pools of compassion.

"I don't know how I would find the time," she whispered softly.

"Why don't you have a think and give me a call. Here's my card with my numbers. It is best to talk in person here at the centre, although, if necessary, we can just talk on the phone." She smiled as she handed Katie a card.

"We can talk about your sleep issues too."

"How did you know?"

"It's my job to see those things. If you must know, you yawn every ten minutes or so. Every week. It's like as soon as you are seated your body screams sleep. Although I bet when you hit the pillow your mind keeps you awake."

"Absolutely."

"If we fix that at least, the rest will feel easier."

Kate smiled a wistful half smile. "It would be wonderful to get a good night's sleep."

"Call me. Let's see what we can do."

"Thank you, I think I will."

Jackie had been standing silently by while this exchange took place. Now she reached over and took Kate's arm.

"Come on we need sleepy time hot chocolate not coffee this evening. And don't worry, I'll nag her till she calls you. You are just what she needs."

Katie glanced sideways at her friend.

"Oh I know you think you run the world very successfully, but even you need a little help every now and then. Come on, my treat tonight and we will make a plan for how you can fit this in."

Smiling Katie kept her arm linked through Jackie's as they set off to the café. First the Good Fairy and now the Cavalry. Perhaps next the Handsome Prince!

Chapter 31

Therapy

July 2019

"What about you?"

"What do you mean? "I've been talking non-stop about me and all my problems!"

"Actually, what you have told me is your mother's problems, your husband's problems and each of your children's problems. Nothing about you."

"But they ARE my problems!" Katie almost shouted. She had been sitting with the therapist for over half an hour and as far as she could tell she had poured her heart out about all the issues she was struggling with. The therapist had stared impassively throughout and was now negating everything Katie had told her. Hadn't she listened at all?

"No, while they impact on you, they are not your problems. Sadly, your mother's dementia is her crisis and your husband's inability to connect with his children is his issue. Each of your children own their choices too, although the little one needs more parental help than the others. I am not saying you can't intervene or help in any of these situations. Nor am I saying it isn't a heavy load you are carrying. However, you have your own underlying needs that aren't being met. If we focus on those you will cope better with the things you can't change.

"My mum won't get better if I don't help." Katie blurted out.

"Is that what you think?"

Katie nodded slightly.

Stephanie, the therapist, leant forward and gently touched her arm. "I'm sure deep down you know this but I am going to say it anyway. You won't win. However hard you try you can't beat Alzheimer's. It is a horrible, often slow, terrible way to die and you cannot stop it. Your mum will decline and she will die. No amount of trying to prevent the inevitable will make any difference."

Katie gulped, her eyes blurred with tears and she looked down at the floor.

"I'm sorry to have put it so bluntly. It is just that at the moment you are harming yourself with false hope. And your children and your marriage. Stop trying to fix what you can't. Let's work on what you can."

"What about Mum? I can't abandon her!"

"Of course not. No one is asking you to do that, that would be cruel. Just remember, while you can make her life a bit more comfortable and support her, you can't fix her. Modify your expectations and recognise that there is only one of you and lots of family. They all need your support. And you need theirs."

"What do you mean?"

"Your husband needs to play his part; we can come to that later. First you can involve your children in helping your mum. Talk to them about how Grandma is getting forgetful. Ask them for help, children tend to respond well to that kind of thing. It makes them feel grown up. They are probably worried about your mum. She is their grandma after all and has been an important figure in their lives. It is up to you how much you tell them, just remember knowing something is better than the unknown. They can make picture labels for rooms or cupboards; the little one might enjoy that. Or walk the dog after school; your middle one loves animals, doesn't she? Involve them in playing memory games with your mum or doing puzzles. All those things will help her and will create memories for them. They will need those when your mum gets worse. To help them cope. And some of it can help you bond with them too. Less tearing you away from them to care for her and more doing it together. Make a set schedule with times you plan to visit her with them, so they are expecting it and give each of them a role in that visit."

"Most of the time I don't know I am going to have to take them. We do that when Mum has an emergency."

"And are any of those actual emergencies?"

"What do you mean?"

"Your mum rings and you go running dragging your children behind you. Yet mostly it is to fix an unbroken TV or something else, that isn't actually an emergency at all. Regular scheduled visits might reduce your mum's anxiety and help reduce those calls too. And get her an easier TV! One that simply turns on at the set and goes straight to BBC1. She will probably never change channels; all she wants it for is company."

Katie smiled. Why had she never thought of that?

"Now we really haven't got on to you, or your marriage. We need to do that next time. Same time next week?"

Katie hadn't intended another session. One to pour it all out and stick a band aid over the issues so she could move on, was all she had had in mind. Tick the therapy box and all that. But…

"Yes please!"

Katie hesitated at the door. She had done what Stephanie had suggested and despite Jack's grumbling about cost had bought her mother a new TV. She had spent hours trawling the internet to find one that was simple, with no success. In the end she had gone into a shop and looked for the oldest assistant she could find, as no young whippersnapper would understand her need. A nice gentleman, clearly working past retirement age, had laughed gently at her explanation of needing a TV her mum could work and found her exactly what she had hoped for. Plug it in, turn it on and up pops the good old Beeb he had said. She put the remote in a drawer and while Joan had protested that it was a silly expense, Katie had managed to convince her it was a gift to replace the one that kept going wrong. She had left Joan watching a gardening programme with a happy smile on her face. A big sign next to the TV pointed to the on switch. Hopefully one problem was now solved.

However, she hadn't talked to her children, nor organised a schedule, nor properly absorbed Stephanie's desperate diagnosis of her mum. She was afraid. Afraid to keep peeling back layers. She needed to fix things, not find out she couldn't.

Stephanie opened the door.

"I thought I heard someone outside. Come on in."

Katie smiled weakly and crossed the threshold.

"I thought we would start with a few practical solutions. I'm guessing I gave you a lot to think about last week and it hasn't been easy?"

"I did change Mum's TV."

"Well done, has it helped?"

"So far, but it was only yesterday."

Stephanie smiled. "That's a good start. I have here the number of a man called Steve Austin."

"The Six Million Dollar Man!" blurted Katie, as a childhood memory pushed to the surface unbidden. "I watched that with Mum. I used to wonder why they couldn't rebuild Dad…" She stopped, stared. "I have never said that to anyone before."

"Do you remember him at all?"

"No, I was a baby when he died. It was always just me and Mum. She never talked about it. We just got on with it. Like people did in those days."

"Is there anyone who could help you find out more about him?"

"No, he was an only child like Mum. I could never bear the sadness on her face if I asked questions. It was so long ago. Too late now to dig into that."

"Perhaps. Although there are ways to investigate our past. However, I don't think that is what matters now. Now we need to deal with some present pressing issues."

Katie nodded.

"The Steve Austin I am talking about runs the local carer's outreach group. It would have been mentioned at the course, but I doubt you have followed that up."

"No, I haven't had time."

"I suggest you make some time this week. He can help you with all kinds of practical things. First, he will help you look into carer's support. There are groups for people who care, and before you say you don't have time, think how much you have gained from your new friend at the course. There is even a respite place for carers to have a free weekend away. Secondly and I think of more interest to you, there are a whole raft of activities your mother can attend. There is a day centre where she can have a hot meal and some social activities. Singing for the brain classes, exercise classes. Lots of things that will benefit her enormously and give you some respite."

"I read about those, in the file when Mum was first diagnosed. I just can't get her there. The day centre is only open on a Friday when I am working. Singing is on a Monday when I have the same issue."

"Steve can help with that too. There is a minibus route that picks up attendees. There's a very small charge. Or there are volunteers who drive people. Talking of volunteers there are friendshipping groups run by local Churches. People who will visit the elderly who live alone and provide a bit of company."

"I'm not sure Mum would like any of this. Won't all those strangers just confuse her?"

"They might. On the other hand, she needs this. Social contact is the best thing for dementia. It will help keep her brain functioning. There are lots of studies that show the positive effects of social contact and specifically singing. She might enjoy herself!"

Still Katie was unconvinced.

"I know it is hard to let go a little. It has been just you and your mum for so very long Katie. Trust me, you both need this. Talk to Steve. You can try these things. If they don't work out, you can stop. Think about it. The fact that there are things on your workdays could be perfect. You won't need to worry about your mum on those days anymore."

"I will call him."

"Good!"

"Now talking of work, I have another thought for you."

"Really? Work is the one thing I am not worried about!"

"I listened really carefully last week Katie. And you are right, on the surface you are not worried about your skills at work. Instead, you are worried about holding onto your job and your family, especially Jack, accepting that you do it."

Katie shook her head at how astute Stephanie was. She was spot on with her analysis.

"Are you doing a good job?"

"Yes, I think so."

"Is your line manager happy with your output?"

Katie grimaced thinking of the deputy head's abrupt manner. And yet since the issue with early mornings had been settled, she had not been unpleasant to deal with. In fact, she had praised Katie for her quality planning and initiatives with the weaker class members."

"Yes, I think she is."

"And are you on top of all your work."

"Yes, I am."

"So, it is time for a little change. You have been there almost a year now and have done a good job. That gives you a little leverage."

"Why do I need that?"

"To change your working week."

"Why?"

"You don't have to take my advice here of course and it may not work out, but here's my assessment of the current situation. The person you job share with was a long-term, full-time member of staff who asked to go part time after she had her first baby, you told me that last week."

Katie nodded, marvelling at how much detail Stephanie had absorbed.

"She chose her working days as the middle of the week leaving you the two dog ends. You start everything off, then she does the middle and you have to pick up the ends. While you leave careful notes at the end of Monday, she just leaves you a pile of "finish off" messes for Friday. And while she has a long weekend both sides your week has no flow to it with Sunday night ruined by the need to prep for Monday."

"That's about right."

"Now you are established, ask for a change. Give two options: Monday and Tuesday or Thursday and Friday. Cite the improvement for the children to have continuity over two days, your chance to complete a section of work. I am sure you can come up with reasons why it would be better for them."

"Yes…it would."

"And for you. It would give you back either Monday to clear up from the weekend or Friday to prepare. Your week would flow better I think."

"You are a genius."

"Thank you," she smiled, "all I am is perspective. It just helps to have someone from the outside look in and assess what is happening. However, my main job is to help you recover yourself. We need to move on and talk about bigger issues."

"Jack?"

"Not exactly. I am not a marriage guidance expert. I can refer you to one if you want, although that would need Jack to join in. In case that never happens, I have some suggestions that might be of use."

Katie smiled and leant forward a little.

"Go on."

Stephanie smiled and looked at Katie. Already she had won her trust and in doing so she could see signs of tension easing around her face and neck. She spent much of her professional life feeling she couldn't fix things; teenagers, adults, even children came to her with woes too big to mend. Although she tried her best and sometimes succeeded. In this case the solutions existed, they were just hard to find if you didn't know where to look. Alzheimer's brought with it such complex difficulties with no medical solution. Therefore, little or no intervention was offered after diagnosis. Instead, carers like Katie were left to pick up the pieces. Depending on the situations in their own lives they often floundered. The courses helped, although participants usually didn't get to one until they had been struggling alone for too long. There should be immediate support, clearly available from the start. While those who had dementia suffered a cruel fate, Stephanie often wondered if the carers suffered worse. This time she was determined to give Katie enough signposts to find her way out of her own personal maze.

"Think back to how you were when you and Jack first got married. How different was your life to before you were married?"

Katie thought carefully and then smiled, "Actually not much changed. I stayed in with Jack rather than went out with him.

Although we did still go out at weekends. I worked full time at the same job. We lived in my flat as it was bigger than his and I carried on the cooking and cleaning as I always had. He did wash up though!"

"You didn't divide up the housework then?"

"No…I didn't even think of it. I just carried on."

"When did the big changes come?"

"When Matt was born. We moved into a maisonette with a little garden. It was nearer to Jack's work. He had a new job and it made sense as I gave up work when Matt was born. We decided that supporting his career was important and that having a parent at home for the baby was ideal. I wanted that role. My mum had to work. Jack's didn't. We both felt it ideal if I was home. Then we both fell in love with our first little house."

"Lots of life changes all at once. How long had you been married by then?"

"Less than a year. I wanted a family quickly. I wanted lots of children. I had been an only child and wanted mine to have siblings. Not that my life wasn't happy growing up, but I felt I missed out."

"Not just on siblings either."

"What do you mean?"

"Your father."

"You don't miss what you never had."

"But you missed siblings."

"Why is this relevant? To now I mean? We were deliriously happy then. Now we aren't."

"We need to unravel how you got from there to now. And already you have given me lots of clues."

"Like what?"

"When you talk of your plans to move or even to support Jack's career and you stay home, you said 'we'. You even repeated twice that you both thought staying home was ideal. Then when you talk about having lots of children and having Matt quickly you switch to 'I'. When we first met and talked, you said Jack had expressed a concern that he was 'pushed out' by the children you insisted on having."

"But…"

"I am not agreeing with him and his way of expressing it was certainly not helpful." Stephanie interjected quickly as Katie's face had darkened. "However, I wonder if your childhood experiences of growing up fatherless have coloured your actions more than you think."

"You think it's my fault Jack neglects his kids?"

"No not at all. I am not a judge who attaches blame. I am just helping you see how things came to be. Then if you want to make changes you can. From my perspective it seems the two of you assigned Jack a role. That of provider. He did that rather well didn't he?"

"Yes, we have a comfortable life."

"It appears neither of you realised he could have had a different part to play until you went back to work. Then suddenly his role needs to change. However, he doesn't have room to manoeuvre as he is already stretched and settled in his role."

"Are you suggesting me working was wrong?" Katie folded her arms and stared.

"No not at all. It just meant some of your other roles slipped a little. You probably could have found an equilibrium if your mother hadn't fallen ill so soon after. That tipped you over the edge. And Jack, so far, doesn't have the tools to help."

"Can he learn them?"

Stephanie smiled. "We can all learn new roles; we just have to want to."

"How does that happen. He clearly doesn't want to."

"Unfortunately, we are running out of time for today and I don't want to finish on an anxious note. However, I will say this. What we need to work out is how to remind Jack of the joys of parenting. And of marriage. To do that you need to find your joy again. If we help you find your old self, he will respond. At least I hope he will. There are no guarantees, but it is a good plan. Over the next week I want you to think of the activities the two of you enjoyed when Matt was little and even before he came along. Make me a list of things you did together, ones Jack enjoyed."

Katie sat very still and looked at her hands.

"It might be a very short list," she murmured.

Chapter 32

Changes

July 2019

Through the next week Katie pushed aside the Jack list and focused on her mother. She rang Steve Austin and found the details of the classes. He was incredibly helpful and put her in touch with a couple nearby. The husband had dementia and his much younger wife was feeling the strain of her husband's diagnosis. She took her Phil to both singing for the brain on Mondays and the day centre on Fridays. She was more than willing to do a little detour to pick up Joan and take her along. In return she asked Katie if they could meet occasionally to "swap notes". It appeared loneliness and dementia go hand in hand Katie thought grimly. She also thought Madeleine and Jackie would get on famously, so decided a girls' night out once a month might do them all good. Maddy jumped at the chance, although Jackie, recognising it as the fantasy it was, suggested a daytime cuppa might be a good first step. They set that up for the following week. Maddy and Phil visited Joan and to Katie's surprise Joan was excited about the prospect of a singing class and even more of a Friday outing for lunch. Katie realised Stephanie had been right. Her mother needed outside stimulus. Was she also right about Jack?

Instead of processing that thought, she set up a meeting with the Head to see if Stephanie had been right about work.

"Katie how nice to see you, what can I do for you?"

"Well, I was wondering. I have been here almost a year now and have really enjoyed my role."

"And we have enjoyed having you, you have done an excellent job by all accounts."

Katie paused. She had rehearsed her lines on the way in that morning. She knew she had to tread carefully but the more she had considered Stephanie's idea the more she had loved it.

"I think there might be a way to improve my work."

"Oh?"

"The thing is, while our job share is working because we both take care to plan around it, I feel I could be more effective if my days were concurrent."

"In what way?"

"As you may know, I have focussed a great deal of energy on the weaker members of my class. Those with learning issues or social back grounds that have meant they were less school ready. Naturally while my interventions are beginning to make a difference, these children are generally slower to complete work. And they are less adaptable. I think if I worked two days in a row, I could get them through their tasks more effectively."

"I see."

"As things stand, the more able cope with the double change over, but I think even they would do better if there were only one hand over in the week."

"I agree."

"Oh….good."

"The question is will Mrs Willows?"

"I don't know, I thought I would run it by you first."

"Very wise. And very well put." The Head smiled, "Although as it happens, we have some movement next year and were thinking of a different role for you. "

"What sort of role?" Katie stuttered.

"Mrs Willows is leaving us at the end of the year. She has struggled with juggling home and school and has decided to be a full-time mother for now. She may have told you she is expecting again, it is no secret, so I am not speaking out of turn. With her leaving we have the opportunity to recruit a new full-time teacher for your class, assuming there are still suitable candidates available as it is late notice.

"Oh…"

"Don't worry, you would still have a job. Unless you wanted full time. We would consider that?"

Reluctantly Katie shook her head, "I really couldn't manage it, much as I would like to."

"Well, how about a role in learning support? You would be responsible for interventions for all the key stage one and foundation children? You would probably need to increase your hours slightly to cover them all. We would be looking at half a day more perhaps? And you could definitely work concurrent days. You would work with Sue who is overall in charge and she would organise some specialist training for you. We have noticed your efforts with these children and think it would be a good fit and Sue needs the help. No pressure though, we could look at a different age group job share for you or even recruit another part-timer and leave you where you are. Although I would prefer to avoid that as like you I think continuity is vital with little ones. This could be a great opportunity for you. It comes with a slight pay increase too. I wasn't going to mention it yet, but as you have asked for a change of sorts what do you think?"

Katie beamed "I think it is perfect!"

It was five minutes before her next appointment, when Katie realised she hadn't written her list about Jack.

Chapter 33

Singing

July 2019

"Hello?" Joan peeped cautiously round her door with the chain still on.

"Hello! We've come to take you to singing."

"Singing? I don't do singing."

Maddy smiled her brightest smile. She had lived with Phil long enough to know that despite Katie's careful introduction and explanation Joan would have no idea who she was.

"I came to see you for a coffee last week. With your daughter Katie. She told me you love to sing so as my husband and I go every week we thought you might like to come too."

"Oh yes of course. Katie sent you!" Joan opened the door and let Maddy through. Maddy marvelled at how easy it was for anyone to talk their way into the home of a dementia sufferer. She was certain Joan still had no idea who she was but, just like Phil would, she was covering up her lack of memory.

"If you get your coat and shoes, we can get going. It's about a half an hour drive."

"Oh yes, of course. Is Katie coming too?"

"Not this time. She asked me to take you for her as she is at work."

"Oh yes. Do I need to pay?"

"There's no charge for the singing but you might like to buy a cup of coffee."

"I will need my handbag then. I'm not sure where I left it."

"Don't worry. I can treat you this week."

"Thank you, that's very kind. Now where did I put my bag?"

Maddy paused, realising the bag was an issue. Just like Phil always took his umbrella. Whatever the weather he had to have it. "OK then she said brightly- let's think; where might it be?"

Joan thought carefully. "I don't know."

Maddy glanced towards the open front door. Phil was sitting quietly in the front seat. She hadn't locked the door and sometimes he got out if she was gone too long, although for now he seemed peaceful enough. Still, she quickly pressed her lock button on her key ring before looking up and down the hall looking for hooks or cupboards.

"Is it in your coat cupboard do you think? Shall we look?"

Joan frowned. She opened the door. Inside was one of Katy's bright labels saying 'coats, hats and shoes.' But no handbag. She shook her head.

"Well at least we found your shoes and coat. Would you like to put those on?" Maddy spotted another small cupboard under the stairs.

"Is your bag in that cupboard?" She pointed.

"Oh no I keep the vacuum in there."

"Shall we check anyway?"

"If you must." Another bright label with a list of cleaning items. Then the boiler with a very firm label over the switch saying not to turn it off. Maddy had to smile while she made a mental note to add some similar labels to her house. It might help Phil be a bit less reliant on her.

"Let's look in your kitchen shall we."

"Oh yes! Katy put it in there. In the top cupboard. So that no one would see it if they came to the door! Here it is!"

Maddy marvelled at the sudden moment of lucidity and added a silent prayer of thanks as she caught sight of Phil trying to open the car door.

Joan looked anxiously around the strange church hall. There were lots of unfamiliar faces, all smiling brightly. Apparently, they were all going to sing to her. Or was she expected to sing to them? Certainly, the friendly woman who had brought her here had talked a lot about singing. She didn't seem to be in charge though. She thought that was a pretty Indian lady who had introduced herself as Priya. It helped that she had given them all big sticky labels with their names on. That felt a bit like being back at school, although it did help her know who was who. She was sitting next to a man called Phil. She thought he came with her in the car with the nice lady who had disappeared. She had helped Joan get a coffee and some biscuits first and made sure she had met Priya. Then with a smile and a wave she had vanished. Joan did hope she was coming back for her.

"Right let's get started, shall we?" said Priya, calling the group to some kind of order. The murmur of voices slowly subsided and all the faces turned expectantly towards their leader.

"I think we have a new lady today. This is Joan everyone, let's please make her feel welcome." Everyone smiled and murmured friendly hellos towards the newcomer. Joan beamed back.

"So, I think we will start with some old music hall favourites. Who remembers "It's a Long Way to Tipperary?""

And so began the most fun hour Joan had had in years. They sang a whole range of songs. Music Hall favourite, hymns, pop and even nursery rhymes. Some she knew and some she didn't. They were told to just la la along if they didn't know the words so that's what she did. There was a flip chart on a board with words on, although she couldn't make them out clearly from her seat. Some people barely sang at all, some just sat and smiled. However, many like Joan raised the roof with their enthusiasm. There was a lovely round lady called Annie who played the piano and sang in a high trilling voice like an old-fashioned school music teacher. Joan loved her. She felt like a child again, taking part in song practice on Friday afternoons. She had loved that bit of school. Memories washed over her and she felt a warm glow of happiness.

Then Priya announced time was up and that their drivers would be waiting in the lobby. Joan panicked slightly. Who was her driver? The man next to her got up and walked towards the lobby. One by one everybody else filed out. Only Joan was left. She looked around anxiously. What should she do now?

"Joan, do you know who is collecting you?" Priya was smiling down at her.

"It might be Katie?" she suggested hopefully.

"Hmm, I think you came in with Phil's wife. Let me go and check, stay there."

At that moment, a bright smiling face that was vaguely familiar came bustling through the door.

"There you are Joan love, I thought I'd lost you when you weren't in the foyer with the others. I've got Phil all seated in the car. Shall we go join him."

Not Katie then, thought Joan sadly, but she got up and followed anyway. The lady seemed to know what she was doing and she did look a bit familiar at least.

"So did you enjoy yourself?" asked Priya.

"Oh yes!" said Joan, "Very much."

"Will you come again?"

"Can I?"

"You can come every week if you want to."

"I would love to! But how will I get here?"

"Don't worry about that, I will bring you with my Phil," said the lady who was steering her out of the door. "I drop the two of you here and go and get my nails done across the road. Do you like the colour?"

Joan smiled and nodded. Whoever this woman was she seemed very kind. She didn't really think gold nails were a good choice, but she thought she had better not say so or she might not get taken home.

"Beautiful," she said, "very shiny."

Maddy beamed as she opened the car door for Joan and helped her in. "We all need a little treat, don't we? Next week I'm having a massage."

"Lovely," smiled Joan.

Later Joan sat quietly in her sitting room. She was vaguely aware she had been out somewhere that day. She remembered a bright shiny lady, some singing and a piano. Oh yes, her teacher had taught them some new songs. What was her name again? Oh yes, Mrs Roberts. She taught the fourth form usually and Joan was second form, but on Fridays they all crowded in the hall together and sang. She loved Friday afternoons.

Chapter 34

Lego

July 2019

Lucy was busy. The holidays had started and she had to sift through all of Matt's discarded Lego to find exactly the right piece. Lego was her new favourite thing. Even better than Barbie or LOL dolls! Matt had been having a clear out and Lucy had pounced on the mountain of old Lego kits. There were all kinds, from Star Wars to Harry Potter to simple Creator mixes. Unfortunately though, Matt had not taken care to keep them separate. Lucy was currently building a giant knight's castle and there was one vital piece of wall missing. She pursed her lips and searched the next box. It had to be there somewhere!

"Lucy! Have you got a minute?"

Mummy's voice wafted up the stairs. She was perhaps old enough to know that "Have you got a minute" really meant "I need to talk to you right now," but Lucy didn't always pick this up. Certainly, on this occasion, she dismissed the distant sound and turned back to her Lego.

"Lucy, I'm calling you!"

Mummy's voice was coming closer as she climbed up the stairs. Still Lucy searched the boxes, brow furrowed with concentration. That annoying piece had to be here somewhere. She couldn't finish the turret without it!

"Lucy! Didn't you hear me? I've been calling you!"

Lucy tore her eyes from the boxes and looked up at her mummy. "I can't find the piece I need," she muttered by way of explanation.

"Never mind that I need to ask you something."

"But it's important. I need the brown piece that fits here, or I can't do this turret right and if that isn't right then this knight doesn't have anywhere to stand," wailed Lucy.

Katie sighed. She needed Lucy to focus on her request yet knowing her younger daughter she realised she wouldn't get her attention until the necessary piece was found.

"Can I help?"

Lucy frowned. Mummy almost never helped with stuff like this. Something must be seriously wrong. She didn't want Mummy to tell her bad stuff. She just wanted to finish her castle.

"OK, it needs to be a brown, 3 brick with this extra bit that moves. See like this one."

For the next 10 minutes the two of them sat, heads bowed searching the boxes until Lucy gave a triumphant shout.

"I've got it!"

She carefully slotted it into place and then picked up the instructions to see what was next.

Katie seized her chance. "Before we go any further Lucy, I need to ask for your help."

Lucy frowned again. Was it going to be tidying up, washing up or even cooking? Those were the things Molly and Matt did for Mummy. All she ever got told was to pick up her toys and Mummy usually ended up helping her as she always had so many out, she couldn't do them all at once. Sometimes she was asked to set the table, although she kept getting the knives and forks the wrong way round and Matt teased her, so Mummy didn't ask her anymore. She put down the Lego instructions and stared at her mother.

"I need your help with Grandma."

Lucy sighed. Another rush across town to fix Grandma's TV. Then again Mummy had got her a new one, hadn't she?

"You know how Grandma is getting forgetful lately? Well apparently, it would be good for her if, once we are all back at school after the holidays, we always visited on the same day and time. And that maybe you can play some games with her to help her remember things."

"Does she like Lego?"

"No…but maybe some puzzles or board games like snakes and ladders."

"They're boring."

"You love puzzles!"

"I did but now I like Lego." Lucy's little chin jutted out defiantly, "Puzzles are boring."

"What about that new pirate ship one. The one you had for your birthday. That isn't boring." Too hard for her mother though, thought Katie. This wasn't going quite how she had hoped.

Lucy put her head on one side reminding Katie of a little bird as she considered this. That was a good puzzle, with loads of interesting characters on it. Maybe she did still like puzzles a bit. just not boring old snakes and ladders.

"Can we play the airport game?"

"What?"

"You know the one where you race across the ocean and up the towers."

"Oh, do we have that?"

"Yes! Mummy don't be silly it was yours!"

"Oh, that game." Recently Jack had been having a bit of a tidy of the garage and had come across a box of old games from Katie's childhood. One relatively obscure one involved racing counters from the top of the Post Office Tower to the Empire State Building and back. The choices of buildings dated it, but Lucy had taken a real shine to it. It was basically just a roll and move game. Her mother should be able to manage that.

"Yes, that would be a good choice. Shall we go after school on Thursdays? You can take the game then."

"OK Mummy."

Katie smiled. Maybe Stephanie's idea would work. Molly had agreed to go to Grandma's every Thursday after school if she was to be allowed to walk Trixie on her own. Then again on Saturday mornings while Matt played football. Matt was more than happy to get himself home on Thursdays and use the spare key hidden in the outside toy box to let himself in. As long as Katie left him some sandwiches in the fridge. Astonishingly Jack was keeping to his football commitment with Matt. Lucy playing games with

Grandma to keep them both amused was the last piece of the puzzle. Then Katie would be able to have a quick tidy of her mum's house or even relax and play too as the cleaner was working out well. She grinned at her youngest child.

"I think that is very grown up of you to help your grandma like that. Now what piece do we need to find next?"

Chapter 35

Therapy Again

July 2019

Katie's third session with Stephanie had not been particularly useful as she hadn't done the preparation Stephanie had wanted. They had chatted positively about the new routines and Katie had told her of the new job offer. However, they had skirted around the marriage problems, with Stephanie summing up the session by saying it was wonderful to hear so much good, although as they only had one more session available, if Katie really wanted to make a difference it would be helpful for her to create the list she had suggested before the next session. Katie had agreed and sat down and pondered it that evening. She was pleased with her efforts and bounced in smiling to the final session, then plonked herself down in the chair opposite her therapist clutching her notebook.

"Someone looks pleased with themselves." Stephanie smiled back.

"I have written my list!"

"Good. Let's hear it then."

"OK, well when we first met, I was very keen on cycling. I used to go out 3 or 4 times a week. Jack bought a bike and started to join me on my weekend ride. We would go to parks or beauty spots and take a picnic to share before we cycled back. I stopped riding in the later stages of my pregnancy, until Matt was able to sit up when we got a bike seat and started the weekend rides again."

"Did you ever restart your personal rides."

"Er…no. I couldn't fit it in. It seemed unfair to take Matt out all weathers just so I could ride and I was so busy coping with a new born. We did have an exercise bike for a bit that I rarely used, so Jack got rid of it in one of the moves.”

“You never thought about Jack minding Matt occasionally so you could ride?”

“Oh gosh no it never crossed my mind!”

“And thereby hangs a tale!”

“Sorry?”

“It is all just part of your family picture. Go on, I will explain when you are done.”

“Well,” started Katie feeling somewhat deflated, “secondly we used to go to the movies a lot.” We both loved big action thrillers.”

“Really?”

“Yes, why do you ask?”

“No reason, what is your favourite.”

“The ‘Die Hard’ franchise I think.”

“OK, I liked the first one too, but the later ones got a bit silly I thought.”

“Oh no I loved the one with his daughter. I know it wasn’t the same high-quality drama, but I loved the car chase and how he just kept coming no matter what, he had to rescue his girl.”

Stephanie smiled and leant forward slightly, “I could spend some time looking into why that affected you so much if you want?”

Katie sat back and folded her hands in her lap.

“You think it’s about my Dad? I never knew him so how could it be? He certainly wasn’t Bruce Willis, nor did he drive a big 10-ton truck off a bridge!”

“I think a lot of your problems stem from your lack of a relationship with your father. But again, let us hold off until you have finished your list. What happened about the movie nights when Matt arrived?”

“Well, we didn’t want to use a babysitter as I wasn’t comfortable leaving him with strangers and as we had moved Mum wasn’t close enough to help. So, we started renting movies to watch at home instead.”

“And how was that?”

Katie scrunched up her face trying to remember.

"Put it differently, do you still do it?"

"No…at least not action movies. We moved on to lots of Disney for the children. When Matt and Molly were old enough, we used to watch a movie with them."

"Quite different to a date night then."

"Yes, good family time."

"Perhaps, do you still do it?"

"No, once Lucy was born it rather fizzled out. Come to think of it, it was the same reason as we stopped our grown-up movies in the first place."

"And what was that?"

"The baby would cry and interrupt and by the time I had resettled him I had missed so much I couldn't pick back up."

"Jack never thought of pressing pause?"

"I always said not to as I would only be a minute."

"It takes a while to feed or change or just resettle a baby, doesn't it?"

"Yes, I suppose it does. Jack got fed up with having to catch me up as I would ask questions."

Katie stopped and looked down at her hands." I am painting quite a bleak picture, aren't I?"

"Yes and no."

"Really?"

"I think you are painting a picture of a young mum who was struggling and didn't know she could ask for help. Also, a husband who had no idea how to offer it."

"And now? Can I learn how to ask now, without making him angry?"

"Yes and no. First you have to understand why you do what you do."

"And why is that?"

"Jack was clearly overindulged by his mother, you told me that yourself, and as you allowed him to continue in that vein he did. He isn't totally to blame; it was the easy option for him, comfortable and familiar. He was used to his whims being met by the woman in his life. You had just taken over from his mother."

"Ouch! I'm not a bit like his mother."

"Maybe not, except you enable Jack to behave as he does. Putting it differently, those early experiences set the pattern. Your needs were continually not being met. He wasn't aware then and so now when you are finally asking for change it is too much for him and he is objecting to the disturbance to his routines."

"You are saying I made us dysfunctional?"

"You aren't to blame; you didn't make anything happen. It is all just consequences of circumstances. You had no idea how a father fits into the picture. You had an outstandingly strong relationship with your mum, so you never felt you missed your dad. However, there are experiences you never had which left gaps. Had you chosen a less self-centred man to marry you might have managed better. Unfortunately, Jack was a product of his upbringing just as much as you."

"Can we fix it?"

"I think so. At least we can make it better. Was there more on your list? Although we have the pattern I think."

"Just one. Holidays. We liked weekends away in the country."

"OK, well I think those might be a bit far off for now. However, we can start to peel back the layers of responsibility and reprogramme you a bit."

"That sounds hard."

"Hopefully not. Hopefully, it will be fun." Stephanie glanced at her watch, "I am afraid we are out of time."

"Oh No! This was my last session and you haven't fixed me!"

"It's Ok. I can squeeze one more in. There is a backup fund if I feel someone needs more than the standard four sessions. After that if you still needed help you could get it privately."

"With you?"

"No, I don't do private. Look let's cross that bridge if we get to it. Same time next week?"

"Yes please."

Chapter 36

Center Parcs

August 2019

It had all been Jack's idea. Probably prompted by Katie's gentle explanation of her final therapy session. Stephanie had encouraged her to look for opportunities to have fun with her family. To stop life being one long round of hard work and tiredness and remember how to enjoy just being with each other. To resurrect some of their old activities together. It seemed Jack had taken the idea literally and one Saturday afternoon he had suggested they book a holiday. Images of sun-drenched golden sand had flashed into Katie's brain. Only for a second. Jack had decided Center Parcs was perfect and she realised quickly as he droned on about all the adventures they would have, that there was no swaying him. He had looked mildly irritated at the look on her face and snapped that he had thought she wanted to go bike riding again. She had smiled and conceded that the children would love it and she would enjoy getting fitter again. She had however expressed concern at leaving her mother for so long. To her absolute amazement he had suggested they bring Joan along.

So here they all were. Staying in a lovely cabin in the woods. Matt had been quad biking and tree climbing. Lucy had tried ballet and tennis and Molly had been excited about the arts and crafts activities. Bikes had been hired for everyone except Joan of course. Matt and the children had raced off excitedly every morning to whatever they had booked. Katie had either followed sedately on the land train with her mother or they had stayed back in the cabin, as watching everyone else have fun was not Katie's idea of a great holiday. She did however have one little indulgence. Jack had splashed out and rented one of the top-notch cabins that had a little sauna at the bottom of its garden area.

Every evening once Lucy was tucked up in bed and Katie had finished the dishes, she would slip down there for a bit of peace and quiet. Jack would be playing board games with the older two and her mother dozing peacefully in an armchair. There had to be a bit of space for her didn't there.

After three days of this, as the others got ready to go to the pool, Katie had rebelled. She was fed up with being left behind. She had packed her mother a swimsuit and today they were going to use it!

And so it was that she was sitting on the edge of the pool with Joan, while Lucy pleaded with her to take her up the top slide.

"Oh come on Mummy! Daddy won't take me up as he says it is too high. Matt and Molly think I could do it and the man says I have to have a grown up for the stairs. You haven't even swum yet, so you have to do something! You might even like it! Oh pleeeease…."

Katie looked at Joan. She was happy enough sitting there dangling her legs in the water. She had refused to get in any further as she said it was cold. It wouldn't be so bad to spend a bit of time with her daughter. There were lifeguards all around and her mum used to swim very well. It wasn't deep where she was.

"Would you mind Mum? If I took Lucy up the slide?"

"Why would I mind?"

"I'd be leaving you here by yourself. Is that OK?"

"Of course! I'm a grown up, aren't I? Now off you go and have some fun. Stop fussing around me."

"C'mon then Lucy, where is this slide?"

By the time they reached the top Katie had relaxed. Lucy had chattered all the way and while the queue was long and slow, Katie had unwound as she basked in the simple pleasure of spending time with her youngest. She had stopped glancing over at Joan whenever the spiral staircase allowed and instead had given herself up to the magic. In the back of her mind, she was planning ways to create more moments like these. Surely her mum didn't need watching every second of the day. She could stay in the cabin with a book once in a while. Katie really needed to connect with her children.

They reached the top. It looked a long way down. The lifeguard explained how they must sit. Lucy was to go first and gleefully climbed into place.

"Wheeeeee," she shrieked as she set off.

Katie was next. With an internal "wheeee" as loud as Lucy's, she felt a rush of adrenaline as she shot down the slide. Bending, twisting and finally splashing she laughed with glee at the bottom. Lucy was waiting for her hopping from one foot to the other.

"Again, Mummy again!"

Katie took her hand and off they went again.

Joan was cold. Her feet were cold, dangling in this water. It was terribly noisy too and more than once laughing children had bumped into her in their rush to get into the water. Then one jumped in much too close and splashed her all over. That was it, she had had enough. Anyway, Katie had disappeared and she needed the toilet. She got up and walked towards the toilet sign. She felt much better away from the noise and the children. As she washed her hands she wondered where her clothes were. She spotted a young woman in a uniform.

"Excuse me but can you help me find my clothes?"

"Of course, let's look at your wristband." Joan removed the bit of rubber on her arm and somehow the smiling young woman used it to find Joan's clothes. All neatly folded in a locker with a towel on top. Joan picked up the towel and wrapped it around her, enjoying its fluffy warmth.

"There's plenty of changing rooms free," said the attendant, "You can use any of the blue ones." When Joan looked confused, she gently led her to a tiny room and placed her clothes neatly on a bench for her.

"There, can you manage from here?" She asked.

"Oh yes," smiled Joan, "Thank you so much for your help."

"No problem, my shift finishes now, but there is plenty of staff around if you need anything else."

Joan gently closed the door behind her and pulled the lock across. Slowly she set about changing out of her swimsuit and putting on her clothes.

After the fifth time the spiral stairs had become too steep for Lucy's little legs and the slide had lost its thrill for Katie. They had bumped into Jack as they set out on the third climb and he had promised to check in on Joan. He had waved a thumbs up at Katie as she splashed into the pool, so she allowed herself to believe he was watching Joan and all was well.

"Mummy can we go under the squirty things now?"

"Yes, I just need to check Grandma is OK."

"Of course she is, she's a grown up, come on Mummy they are only on for a minute!"

"I know but…" Lucy wasn't listening and had headed off towards the deep water where all kinds of exciting things were happening. And all kinds of hidden dangers for an over excited young child lurked, thought Katie as she glanced desperately about, hoping to spot Jack or Matt to take over with Lucy. But the pool was packed and she had to rush to stop Lucy leaping into the waves out of her depth. Surely her mum would still be sitting where she had left her?

When the waves and water cannon had finally stopped, Katie was determined to check on Joan. She grabbed Lucy's hand and promising her another go on the slide afterwards; she dragged her towards where Joan had been sitting.

Joan had dressed and was feeling much better. She decided to head off back to the cabin. She saw a sign marked exit and followed it out. She wasn't sure which way to go but as she anxiously looked around, she spotted an arrow on the ground that pointed left, so she headed off to the left. To her delight the land train was parked a few metres on. She had been on that with Katie! She climbed on and sat down smiling at the driver.

"Where are you going?" he asked.

"Back to my room," said Joan.

"Where is that?"

"In the cabin in the woods!"

"Do you want Maple, Birch, Oak or Pine?"

"Oak please!"

"Okey dokey, then off we go."

Joan smiled benevolently at the driver. She wondered why she had to choose a tree, but oaks were her favourites, so big and strong. She would quite like to see some oak trees.

Katie had dragged Lucy round every inch of the pool area and Lucy was starting to cry when she finally found Jack with Molly and Matt.

"Mum's disappeared! I thought she was with you!" exclaimed Katie.

"You asked me to check on her that's all," retorted Jack.

"I thought you would stay with her!"

"You didn't ask me to and Molly wanted to go in the waves and you don't like her doing that by herself! What were you doing leaving her alone like that?"

"Looking after Lucy!" I needed a bit of fun; I've been stuck with Mum all week!"

"She's your mum!"

"Yes, but you said to bring her."

"Only because you wouldn't come otherwise."

Lucy started to wail; she didn't like their raised voices. Molly's lip trembled.

Matt intervened, "Mum, Dad this isn't helping us find Grandma. Why don't you girls go and get changed together. Dad and I will do a last look around the pool and speak to the lifeguards. Mum, go and ask some of staff around if anyone has seen her."

Blinking at the sudden grown-up sense coming from her son, Katie watched the girls trot off obediently hand in hand, calling after them to them to sit on the bench and wait for her when they were ready. Then she headed towards the nearest uniformed youngster.

"She probably just got bored and went for a cup of tea," he said helpfully.

"In her swimsuit!"

"I imagine she got changed first," said the bemused young man.

Too worried to be bothered to explain how her mother would never find the changing rooms, let alone locate her own clothes, she left him and headed to the cubicles anyway. Maybe by some miracle Joan would be there.

Joan was happily watching the world go by. She loved this little train trundling slowly through the woods and chatted happily to whoever got on and sat in front of her. Most people only stayed a little while, but they were all lovely and friendly. Now she was the only one left as the driver pulled up to the latest stop. He turned and looked surprised to see her.

"I thought you wanted Oak?"

"Did I?"

"Well, that's what you said."

"Never mind I am sure I can see some other trees just as lovely here."

"Ok, but it is a long walk back to Oak, if that's where you are staying?"

"Oh no we are staying in a cabin!"

"Um, yes but in Oak?"

"No, it's not a treehouse, it's a cabin," Joan looked around and saw some cabins. They looked like the one she was staying in, didn't they? "We're in that one over there," she pointed vaguely as she smiled and got off the train.

"If you are sure, it's just this is Maple and…"

"Thank you for a lovely ride, I've had such a nice time, but I must get on, Katie will be wondering where I am."

The driver watched as Joan strode purposefully towards the cabins. Something didn't seem right, but he couldn't really do anything could he? Perhaps he should go after her and just see her into her cabin? He started to get up, then a family climbed aboard. He glanced over towards Joan. She seemed to know where she was going. He smiled at the newcomers, started his engine and drove away.

Joan tried the door of the first cabin she came to. It was locked. She tried the next, same thing. The third one opened and she walked on in. A strange woman shrieked, "Who are you!" and she stumbled back out muttering "I'm terribly sorry." She looked around. This was all wrong. Where was she and where was Katie? She didn't like it in this strange place. Maybe she had better just go home. She started to walk.

The pool manager had reassured Katie that if her mother had fallen in the water the lifeguards would have spotted her. Even so he had sent extra staff in to do a sweep of the area. He also put a call out for Joan over the tanoy system but to no avail. By then the whole family were gathered in his office.

"I think it would be wise for your son to take the little ones back to your cabin. I know you think it unlikely, but your mother may have found her way there. I'll call security and tell them we have a lost, vulnerable adult. They will know how to find her. Do you have a picture on your phone at all?"

Katie nodded and showed him a shot from the day before. Joan was beaming in a bright red top and floppy sunhat as she watched Lucy playing on a swing.

"One without a hat maybe?"

She scrolled back to find one, as Jack gave Matt some money for ice creams and told him firmly to keep the girls in the cabin until they got back. He was of course to phone them if Joan turned up.

Six security men arrived and started copying the photo. They spoke rapidly into radios, alerting staff all over the complex that Joan was missing. The lakeside staff were instructed to do a sweep along the beach area which terrified Katie, although rationally she couldn't believe her mother would have walked that far. Then again, she didn't think she would have left the pool.

Jack kept pacing up and down. Katie just wished he would go back to the cabin. He wasn't helping.

"Right, I think that's all we need from you my dear," said the chief security man. "Don't worry this is a totally secure site. She can't leave without someone spotting her and as no one leaves on foot the security on the gate would be suspicious if she tried. They all have her photo now so will be on the lookout. Staff all over the complex know to watch out for her. We will find her, it's just a matter of time."

Katie smiled weakly. There was a reel of disasters running in her head; Joan fallen in the lake, Joan knocked over by a bike, Joan in the woods falling over a tree root, Joan stumbling around lost and frightened. Why oh why had she left her!

"Come on Katie, let's go and check on the kids. Let the men do their job."

"You go, I am going to look around myself. She is probably nearby after all."

"We've covered all these shops and cafés already," said the security man. "Your husband is right. Go be with your children. They are probably frightened a bit too. They need their mum. I promise we will find her."

Reluctantly Katie went.

Jack had suggested a board game to pass the time. The children chose Cluedo. He partnered Lucy and took on the other two. Katie watched, wishing she could join in, while the children shrieked with delight as Miss Scarlett was stranded in the living room when she wanted to reach the hall and candlesticks and wrenches were declared unlikely murder weapons. She was too distracted to play and passed the time vaguely preparing a salad and some jacket potatoes for dinner. She knew her family would want to eat even if her stomach was so fiercely knotted it felt like nothing would ever be allowed in it again. The kitchen area looked out over the woods, meaning she kept scanning the horizon for her mother. Every few minutes she would walk across to the living room, ostensibly to check on the game and make some remark to her family, yet really so she could look out of the front window.

"Katie do stop pacing! It isn't helping and it's making us all nervous." Jack put his cards down in frustration.

"I can't see anything here but a family playing a nice game," hissed Katie.

"What else can we do? We were told to wait. The children can't just sit and worry- or pace!" Jack was talking in that condescending tone that drove her crazy. He was right though; she didn't want the children to be upset.

"I'm going to go outside and take a look around this area. I will have my phone so you can ring me if she turns up. You stay here with the children; they seem happy enough."

"If you must."

Katie walked to the door and put on her shoes. As she went to go, Lucy leapt out of her seat and flung herself at her mother grabbing her tightly.

"Don't go Mummy," she whispered, "I don't want you to get lost too."

Katie crouched down and looked into her little girl's eyes. Tears were brimming and she still clung to her mother.

"I won't get lost sweetheart. Grandma is only lost because her memory doesn't work very well anymore so she doesn't know where she is."

"But you might forget too."

"I promise I won't." Lucy still held onto her mother as the tears started to fall.

"Mummy…." she whispered, "I'm sorry."

"What for sweetheart? You haven't done anything wrong."

"Grandma got lost because you were with me."

Katie hugged her little girl tight and kissed the top of her head.

"Oh Lucy I am supposed to be with you! You are my little girl and we were having a lovely time. Grandma was in a safe place which she chose to leave. She got herself lost. You didn't. Now wipe your eyes and let's go back to the game. I have a feeling Mrs White is the culprit. Let's see if I am right!"

Lucy sniffed and followed her mother back to the table. Jack nodded imperceptibly as Katie sat down with Lucy on her lap and took over his cards. Glancing back to reassure himself all was well, he went to the door, pulled on his shoes and quietly cursing the day he invited his mother-in-law along on their holiday, slipped out to join the search.

He needn't have bothered. Half an hour later a beaming Joan was returned to the flat, sweeping in with a smile and a story of having a lovely walk and meeting a kind policeman who walked back with her. The security man pulled Katie to one side.

"We had a tip off she was up in the Maple area. A land train driver saw the alert and remembered an old lady who had seemed a bit confused riding round and round on his train. Apparently, she insisted her cabin was up there when previously she had said Oak, so he let her off and thought nothing more of it until he saw the alert over the system. It's a big area but we were helped by a family who said she had wandered into their cabin. She seemed very confused, until we said we would take her to Katie, when she brightened up. We had first aid check her over. Apart from a small scrape on her knee which she can't remember doing, she seems fine. Except for the obvious of course."

Katie smiled weakly and thanked him profusely.

"We are just doing our job. We get quite a few lost grannies every year. It is easier than children as they tend to move slower. I wouldn't leave her alone if you can avoid it though. Just in case. I wouldn't want you to be so worried again."

"Don't worry I won't," said Katie fervently.

"Enjoy the rest of your holiday," added the security man as he went towards the door.

How? Thought Katie grimly.

Chapter 37

New Shoes

September 2019

Katie was aware that the rest of the school break had not been ideal for her children. Matt was alright; he had taken to catching the bus to see his mates every day. She knew he was old enough, although her heart ached to spend more time with her oldest. She felt he was slipping away from her too fast. The girls had a few playdates each, then the rest of the time they had to fit in with Katie's determination to ensure her mother was safe. All her mother's carefully coordinated activities had stopped for August and even the cleaner was on holiday.

It was fine on sunny days. She would pile them into the car, giving them both a kindle to keep them amused for the journey. At first, they obediently looked at books she had downloaded, but after a week or so they were playing on mindless apps. She excused this to herself with "it's only 20 minutes it won't hurt". It was in fact 20 minutes each way and often Lucy didn't lift her head from hers when they arrived, especially if Joan needed help with something. Then Lucy would stay quietly playing on it in a corner. Molly liked to help and would carefully dust or tidy for her grandma.

Then they would head off to the park. Molly loved the dog and would spend much of her time trying to coax a bemused Trixie to chase a ball or a stick. Lucy would play on the swings and slides while Katie and her mother sat on a bench and chatted. At least Joan talked and Katie listened. She had noticed how her mother increasingly repeated the same few stories over and over. Her unique habit of commenting on strangers as though she knew them, had also become more marked. That same man was always riding his bike, that same mother had been there with her children the day before and so on. "That same mother" is me thought Katie ruefully. Every day.

Rainy days were worse. Then she would pull out a craft activity for the girls to do when they visited Joan. That worked with Molly, but not Lucy who was either quickly bored or needed help. She would whine and complain until Joan would put the TV on for her. Smiling that it was OK "just this once". Katie hated her child watching so much television. There just weren't a lot of options. They sometimes pulled out a board game or puzzle like in term time visits, although Katie didn't want to overdo them as she knew she would need them when they went back to school. Taking Joan anywhere else was fraught with difficulties Katie couldn't face. Sometimes they would reverse the process and take Joan home with them. At least then the girls had all their toys to play with. Then that meant twice as much time in the car for the girls with picking her up and taking her back.

All in all, Katie was glad when it was time for everyone to head back to school. Just one thing to do first. Everyone needed new school shoes.

Lucy was so bored and fed up. Why did she have to go last? First Matt had scowled his way through his fitting for sensible shoes, followed by new trainers and his favourite; football boots. He had tried on no less than six pairs until he was happy. Six! And Lucy had to just sit there and watch. Mummy had left her kindle in the car. He had then been allowed off to look around the other shops on his own, he hadn't had to wait for her and Molly to have their turn. Lucy wanted to go next, but Mummy had picked Molly. Molly had sat there, little Miss Perfect, while the assistant measured and then produced three styles of gorgeous patent leather shoes with shiny buckles. Molly had picked ones with flowers on them and a unicorn printed on the base. Lucy loved them and wanted some the same. Molly had pink trainers too which flashed as she ran. Lucy coveted those most of all.

Afterwards Molly was allowed to go to Claires next door and choose a new hairband. Mummy had given her money to pay for it as well. While she Lucy, had to just sit and go last. The assistant had measured her feet and declared them "very wide". She didn't know what that meant but she knew which shoes she wanted when she was asked. She wanted the same as Molly.

Horrifically Mummy had said no. Lucy had to have Velcro as she couldn't manage buckles yet. Well, how did Mummy know if she hadn't let her try yet? Worse Mummy had said she couldn't have shiny ones as Lucy was "hard on her shoes" whatever that meant and would scuff them. Lucy had pleaded with Mummy, but Mummy wasn't listening. They hadn't even got to trainers yet, although by now she was pretty sure Mummy would have an excuse not to get her the flashing ones. Lucy was cross. She folded her arms and glared at her mother.

"Oh do be a good girl Lucy, your mummy has to get us all new shoes." Grandma was smiling at her. Lucy turned her hard little stare on her grandmother.

"It's not fair, I want shiny ones with buckles like Molly."

"Well, that's easy," said Joan, "She can have them can't she Katie?"

"No," said Katie firmly.

"Why ever not?"

"Because she can't do buckles and she will ruin them in five minutes with her antics. Now come on Lucy try these ones on?"

"No."

Lucy could see her mother was getting very cross. Grandma seemed to be on her side. Maybe Grandma could convince Mummy she was big enough to try buckles. Maybe Grandma would even help her learn. Struck by this thought Lucy turned to Joan.

"Grandma, if I got buckles would you help me learn how to do them?"

"Of course I would sweetheart, we could practice every day!"

Lucy turned to her mother, eyes shining in triumph.

"See Mummy, Grandma will help me!"

Katie looked from one to the other. Her youngest daughter and her mother both looking at her eagerly with hopeful smiles. The thought of early mornings with Lucy struggling to do up buckles and how she would end up doing them for her so they could leave on time flashed through her mind. Followed by images of the notes home she would get about PE and how her daughter needed to manage her own shoes. No, she determined. No way. She decided to divide and rule.

"Mum can you just go to the door and see if Molly is on her way back yet? Don't go out the door though, just look down the street." She hadn't liked sending Molly out on her own, but it was only the shop next door and she had wanted to focus on Lucy. Her feet were always hard to fit. Also, taking Lucy and her mother into Claires would have been a nightmare. Lucy always wanted an impossible range of ribbons and bows that she lost within days and her mother inexplicably kept picking things up and debating what would suit her. Molly would come back safely, with a sensible hairband, wouldn't she?

"Lucy sweetheart we need to get Velcro just one more time. Then you can be quick for PE."

"I don't want Velcro. Velcro is for babies!"

"No, it's not! Grandma has Velcro."

"Babies and old ladies then!"

Katie tried another tack.

"How about the assistant sees what she has in your size? There might be something lovely."

She turned to the lady helping them who was listening intently.

"I need some idea of what style you want," she smiled, "We have a lot of shoes."

"Buckles and shiny." said Lucy.

"Velcro and matt." said mum. "Blue or black only," she added as an afterthought. The school only allowed blue or black.

The assistant looked from the firm looking lady to the cross little girl and turned towards the stockroom.

Katie glanced at her watch. They had already been in the shop an hour. They had been number 21 in the queue and only waited fifteen minutes to be seen. Although that had been long enough with them all twitching and complaining. She glanced at the flashing number. It was now showing 26. That meant the other assistant had dealt with 5 families while she had been there. She looked around the shop. There were at least another five waiting.

She looked back to the door where her mother had been two seconds ago. Where was she?

"Sit there Lucy and don't move!"

She rushed to the door her heart thumping. She had only glanced away for a second! Joan couldn't have gone far! Molly was at the door.

"Hello Mum I got the hairband - look. And here's your change."

"Where's Grandma?"

"She wasn't with me," a bemused Molly replied.

"Sorry, I know, I asked her to stand at the door to see if you were coming as you were ages and now she's disappeared. Did you see her?"

"There was a long queue I had to wait."

"I know I'm not cross with you; I just need to find Grandma." Katie recognised the fear in Molly's voice. "Sorry sweetheart, you did really well."

Molly smiled at the praise, while a gentle frown creased her face. "Do you want me to go and look for her?"

Katie glanced back at Lucy. The assistant had returned with a pile of boxes. She realised she would have to waste precious seconds telling her they would have to leave and come back. Yet what else could she do. She felt herself panicking. It was just like Center Parcs all over again. Why oh why had she told her mum to move?

"I found some!"

Katie spun round to see a smiling Joan.

"Oh Mum you're safe!"

"Of course I am, I'm in a shoe shop!" Joan laughed.

Katie grabbed her hand and started to lead her back to Lucy. The assistant was looking decidedly fed up. Lucy was still scowling. Or was she? Actually, she looked rather smug. In fact, so did the assistant? Something wasn't right.

Katie sat down with a thud. She couldn't do this anymore. However, Lucy still needed new shoes. She tried to pull a smile back onto her face; it presented more like a grimace.

"What do we have for Lucy to try?"

The assistant smiled back at her.

"Well while you weren't here, I had a little chat with your daughter. It appears she wants the same trainers as your other daughter. I have those in her size. I thought maybe if we tried those first, she might be happier to try your choice of shoes."

Katie shook herself into the present. This might work!

"And did they fit?"

"Perfectly."

"So, shoes….?"

Again, the assistant smiled. "We found a compromise. These aren't patent leather, but they do have a mermaid on the bottom and this cute little flower attached to the Velcro strap. Lucy likes those."

"Do they fit?"

"Yes they do! They are especially designed for little girls with wide feet."

Katie wanted to hug her but instead she whispered softly, "Thank you," followed by, "Do you like them Lucy?"

"Yes I do Mummy!"

"So we are all done. Thank goodness for that!"

"What about me?"

Katie turned back to her mother who she realised was standing there clutching a pair of green lace up shoes.

"What do you mean? You don't need new shoes."

"You told me to go and look for some. I like these ones. Do you have them in my size?"

Katie caught the assistant's eye. She was struggling to suppress a giggle. Katie suddenly felt a huge wave of something swell inside her. Whether it was laughter, relief or frustration, she didn't know but she knew it was about to explode out of her. She forced it back down. She looked at her mother's expectant face, Molly's worried one and Lucy's oh no I can't wait another second in this place one and realised she had about ten seconds to settle this all down.

"Right then Mum, we will need to go to the grown up's department for those. Thank you," she smiled at the assistant, "you have been extraordinarily helpful. Girls pick up your new shoes and let's go pay. Then Grandma can try on hers and after that we will all go and get ice cream."

Everyone seemed to be OK with that idea, so Katie started to usher them forwards.

"I don't know how you did it but thank you." She murmured to the assistant.

"Experience," smiled her saviour and nodded towards Joan. "I don't know how you do it though. That must be so hard to manage. I hope the rest of the day gets easier."

Katie swallowed a huge lump and blinked rapidly.

"Thank you." She whispered back.

Chapter 38

Dancing with Katy

September 2019

Katy knocked tentatively at the door. She hadn't seen much of her friend over the long summer break and was worried she would have been forgotten. A radio was blasting from somewhere in the house. Realising Joan wouldn't hear her above the racket she knocked again, louder this time. The music played on and no one came although the little dog barked. She waited, clutching the tray of old-fashioned fairy cakes she had made after remembering Joan had informed her modern cupcakes weren't as nice as the ones her mother made. She had searched for a recipe online and was quite proud of how they had turned out. She would never eat a dozen alone though and thought they would be the perfect ice breaker. She hesitated, considering leaving, then just as she turned to go the door burst open.

"Katy how wonderful! Have you come to dance?"

"Erm, well I suppose I can."

"Great! Come on in! I'm practicing for my show you know."

Katie followed Joan through to the living room where the music had paused for an insurance advert. Joan frowned at it.

"Where's it gone? I was working on my waltz. I don't want all this talking."

"It will come back in a moment. Shall I turn it down while he talks?"

"Oh yes please. Ooh cakes how lovely. Shall I pop the kettle on?"

Together they made tea and sat companionably in the living room. The radio hummed softly in the background as Joan focussed on demolishing the cakes.

"These are delicious. Did you make them? They are just like the ones my mother used to make. Light and fluffy and not too much icing. Perfect. Not like those newfangled ones."

"Yes, I did thank you. I'm glad you like them so much. I thought you might save one or two for your grandchildren."

Joan paused as she reached for her fourth cake.

"Yes, I probably should. I'll just have this one."

Katy sipped her tea and watched her friend happily munching. It was lovely to feel she could brighten someone's day so easily.

"What made you want to dance today, Joan?"

"Dance?"

"You said you were practicing when I arrived?"

"Oh, yes. Well, I used to dance in competitions you know. I was very good. Especially the waltz. I met my husband on the dance floor. He loved to waltz. I don't do it now though. I've no one to dance with."

Katy swallowed, realising the radio had simply triggered an old memory and Joan had felt compelled to react.

"Would you like to dance some more? I could try to do it with you. I had lessons when I was a little girl. I can do a simple waltz."

"It's not the right music now." replied Joan sadly. The radio had moved on to a symphonic piece not at all suitable for dancing.

Katie smiled, switched it off altogether and whipped out her phone.

"Some modern things are good," she grinned. "I have some Strauss on here that I like to listen to when I'm marking. I find it more uplifting than pop!"

Joan grinned too as Katy turned the sound up high and they stood facing each other.

"I'll be the man," said Joan. "That means I'll lead. Now you put your hands here. You have to hold your head like so." Katy did as she was told, feeling slightly awkward as she held the old lady's waist.

"Now it's just one two three, one two three…."

They started slowly, then as Katy relaxed and Joan remembered, they started to twirl and swirl around the room.

Joan was lost in her past as the music played on and Katy caught the joy of it. Round and round they went until suddenly Joan faltered and stopped.

"I'm quite puffed. I think I need to sit down."

Katy helped her to a chair.

"Would you like another cup of tea?"

"Oh yes please. And maybe one of those delicious looking cakes. Did you make them?"

Chapter 39

What If?

October 2019

Joan was waiting by the door. She wasn't quite sure what she was waiting for, but she knew there must be something. Every day there was something now. Katie had "arranged" things. Joan was getting a bit tired of being "arranged". She wanted to just sit quietly for a day. She looked anxiously out of the window to see who was going to appear today. There was a rather loud lady and a quiet man who took her places. Sometimes to eat and sometimes there was singing. She liked singing. Although she preferred dancing. She used to do competitions once. Sometimes that felt like yesterday, although she knew it couldn't be. She loved the swish of a taffeta ballgown as she sashayed across the floor. She tried to get Katie to practice with her once, but she was very grumpy about it. Katie was always so rushed! Katy was happy to dance with her though. She found old fashioned music on her phone for them and they practiced a waltz or two. What fun!

Worst of Katie's arrangements was the lady who came and cleaned. She didn't like that so much. Having a stranger move all her things about. She wanted it to stop but Katie insisted. Katie was getting a bit bossy! Most of all she liked it when Lucy came. Lucy would sit and play games with her. Lucy didn't mind if she got it wrong. She would just say "Oh Grandma!" and laugh and they would start over.

Trixie barked. Was someone coming? No sign. Poor Trixie, she wanted her walk. Joan couldn't go in case today's Someone came. She looked down as the eager little dog wagged her tail furiously.

"Come on Trixie, let's get your lead. I don't want to go anywhere today anyway."

Katie dismissed her pupils for playtime, quietly helping the smaller children on with their coats. Her new role meant more planning and recording and she was looking forward to a break time cuppa and a chance to get ahead, making sure she wouldn't have too much for the weekend. Before she headed to the staffroom, she quickly checked her phone. Two voicemails and five texts. She checked who left the voicemails first seeing that both were Maddy. Probably about their planned catch up later that week. The planning beckoned as she scrolled the texts, dismissing the ones from Jack to deal with later. Then her stomach lurched as she spotted one from Maddy. 'CALL ME', it said. She did.

"I only have a moment, what's up?"

"I went to pick up your mum today for lunch club and she didn't answer the door. I went round the back but no sign of her. I thought you should know."

Katie frowned. Was there something wrong or had her mum simply forgotten Maddy was coming today.

"Thanks Maddy. I will pop over later and see what's up. In the meantime, I will call her. She probably forgot you were coming."

"I know, goes with the territory I'm afraid."

"Was the dog barking by any chance?"

"No...now you mention it... I don't think she was."

"Mum probably took her out then. Not to worry. Sorry she wasted your time."

"Oh, it's no problem. See you later."

Katie hung up and quickly pressed her mother's number. She let it ring a long while, yet no one picked up. She shook her head to release the tension and went on to get her cup of tea. She was not going to panic. Her mum was probably just walking the dog.

Joan had been for a lovely walk and was settling down for a nice tea and biscuits when the phone started ringing. She was comfortable and didn't feel like getting up to answer it. She left it ringing. She popped her new TV on instead. A gardening programme. Lovely!

Katie put her phone back in her bag again. It was lunchtime now and she was starting to worry. Joan was either on a very long walk or something else had happened. Images of her mum lying at the bottom of the stairs flashed in her brain. Or knocked over by a car, or …. She shook herself. She had to get on with her sewing club. She would just ring again in afternoon break.

Joan opened the fridge. All that she could see was those horrible microwave meals Katie insisted on having delivered. She was bored of those. She fancied some chocolate. She put her shoes and coat on, picked up her bag and slipped out to the shops. As she closed the door behind her the phone started to ring. Never mind, probably just one of those charities calling for money. They rang every day now. So many causes she was supposed to help with. Not today though. She wanted some chocolate.

Katie's hands shook as she turned off her phone. What on earth was going on. One more hour and then she could dash to her mother's house. What about the children? She hesitated and then rang the girls' school. They could stay later at after school club tonight. It would be better they weren't with her if something was wrong with their grandma. And she would get to Joan quicker if she didn't go to collect them first. She could text Matt on his new mobile. He had his key and could make himself a snack. Her dinner plans would be messed up as she wouldn't have time to cook the special fish dish she had promised Jack. She would pull something out of the freezer instead. She had to check on her mum.

Lucy was tired. She wanted to go home not to after school club at all and Mummy should be here by now. Where was her mummy? The teacher had just said she would be late. But why? She walked head down across the hall and sat on a chair. She didn't want to play. She wanted to go home.

Joan was just tucking into her fourth Viennese fancy. They had been on special offer and she couldn't resist. Yummy. The doorbell rang. She sighed. She really didn't want to see anyone today. She decided to just ignore it.

"Mum!" Mum! Are you there?" Someone was banging on the back door and shouting. Trixie was yapping horribly so Joan couldn't make out what they were saying. Joan didn't like the idea of opening the door to such loudness. She shrunk back into her chair and stayed still.

Katie felt sick. Should she call the police? Break the door down herself? She could break a window to get in. Not at the back though, Trixie might get hurt by the glass. She would go round the side to the little study window. She looked round for a stone big enough to smash a hole. She wrapped her cardigan around her hand to protect it, closed her eyes and crash!

Joan screamed. Someone was breaking in. She looked around wildly. Then picked up a little stool. If the intruder came in her living room, she would throw it at them.

Katie's arm was bleeding slightly from where she had reached through to open the window. She had squeezed herself in and was looking around frantically. Where would her mum be? She checked the kitchen first. Nothing. She opened the living room door. Her eyes stared in shock as the stool flew into her face.

Katie was sitting on the sofa. She had an ice pack for her bump and her heart rate was starting to return to normal. Joan looked at her fiercely.

"Why did you break in my house?"

"I thought you were hurt Mum."

"But why? I was just eating Viennese fancies! I would have given you one, but I shan't now!"

"You didn't open the door."

"I didn't know it was you."

"But how would you know without answering it. I called out."

"You made Trixie bark with all that banging. I couldn't hear you. I've had a lovely quiet day today with none of your organising me and I didn't want to be disturbed!" Joan crossed her arms belligerently.

"You never answered your phone all day."

"I don't have to do what you want all the time! I'm a grown up! Please Katie, leave me in peace."

"You hit me with a stool."

"I thought you were a robber."

"Oh Mum." Katie's head throbbed and her eyes welled with tears. Her mum was staring at her crossly like she was somehow in the wrong. Yet she had been so afraid for her. So frightened she was hurt. There was no way of explaining it, Joan was clearly not going to understand.

"I'm going now Mum. I need to get the children. I will arrange for someone to come and mend your window. Don't go in there for now as there is glass everywhere."

"I will have to sweep it up."

Katie sighed, "No I will do it. And I'll put something over the break to stop rain getting in until it is fixed. I'm sorry Mum."

Joan softened.

"Honestly Katie I don't know what got into you. Would you like a Viennese fancy after all?"

Lucy put the last of the unicorns back into the box. She and Molly were the only ones left. The lady in charge had asked them to help tidy up. Still Mummy hadn't come. She looked at her sister with frightened eyes.

"Where's Mummy?"

Molly shrugged. She didn't know either. She looked up at the lady in charge who was clearly fed up and not inclined to be comforting. After all it was past the end of the day and she wanted to go home. Didn't some people realise it was Friday?

"Lucy! Molly! I'm so sorry."

Lucy hurled herself at her mother and burst into angry tears.

"Why did you leave us so long Mummy, why?"

Katie hugged her little girl tight, confused by the tears.

"Did something happen Mrs Roberts? To upset Lucy?"

"Just you not turning up till late on a Friday I expect." She muttered gruffy.

"But Lucy you love after school club?"

"I love you more."

Holding tight to each of her daughters Katie turned for the door. Dinner was going to be take away and she was expecting a lot of eye rolling and worse from Jack. Matt had probably stuffed himself with biscuits by now. She had been such an idiot. But what if?

Chapter 40

The Garage

October 2019

Katie loved her new role. Monitoring the children with learning difficulties and ensuring they received the support they needed was a rewarding if time consuming challenge. There was a great deal of paperwork to do, although this year she was given time during the school day for that and her lesson preparation. This was a novelty she had never experienced as a part time teacher. Despite the rules that stated they should have proportional planning times, it was rarely given in small schools like hers, with such limited staffing and budgets.

Teaching was increasingly a job of two halves. The joyous part of dealing with children and the tedious part of filling in forms. Still, she was coping and the new hours worked well. Her change of days had also meant Molly could stop after school club one evening and instead attend the craft club she had longed to join. She hadn't been able to as it would have meant Katie had to pick her and Lucy up at different times. In another life when her mother was well, that would have been possible. Instead, pushing the guilt to one side and letting uncomplaining Molly miss out had been easier, in case they had had to squeeze in an after school trip to Joan's too.

Those days were gone. If Katie was working, her mother was going to clubs or the day centre. On days she wasn't, Katie spent her daytimes with her and the evenings with her children. The cleaner was back and doing both houses which took another strain from Katie's shoulders. The summer had been one thing; term time had to be different. She always rang her mother around

9pm after the children were in bed to remind her to let the dog out for a bit then lock the doors and go to bed. Those chats sometimes tried Jack's patience, although it meant Katie went to bed peacefully believing her mum safe and well.

The difficult days were the weekends. Either she went to collect Joan both days and kept her with them, or she ended up running back and forth. It was certainly easier just to collect her first thing and trail her around with them all day. She knew it frustrated Jack and limited what they could do. However, otherwise, she would be dashing back and forth to do meals and ensure her mother was safe. Matt took himself to football these days and while Katie felt a bit guilty that neither of them watched every match, it certainly reduced the problems of keeping the girls happy on the side lines or of Jack complaining he had missed out on his quiet Saturday mornings.

Washing was shovelled in and out of machines at an alarming rate and ironing done when the children went to bed. Katie was grateful for the cleaner who tackled the bigger jobs on Mondays. However, she still found herself cleaning up behind the children on a Sunday afternoon as she couldn't stand the mess. The girls were often happy to just play at home and Joan enjoyed watching them. Keep it simple the course had taught her. Often dementia sufferers just like to be with someone they love. They don't need to be rushing about. Jack spent more and more time brooding behind his paper or oddly disappearing to the room over the garage. She didn't ask.

Trixie was becoming an increasing worry that Katie kept trying to ignore. She knew Joan often forgot to feed her, despite the carefully weighed out individual portions of food Katie prepared for her each week and left in labelled bags. Some were not used at all, some on the wrong days and sometimes Joan would feed her random scraps or inexplicably cornflakes and milk. Trixie's once immaculate coat looked matted and her toilet habits were not so reliable. Katie knew the little dog still barked to go out; Joan simply didn't always respond. Nor did Joan walk her further than the end of the road alone anymore. She seemed to have accepted that she would not find her way home. On Katie's visit days she would take them both out and the little dog loved it when Molly came to play. More and more she spent hours alone at home. Katie knew that could not go on. She had given a neighbour a key and asked her to let Trixie out and feed her on Saturdays and Sundays. However, she wasn't very reliable and often they returned home to find Trixie hungry and forlorn with a puddle by the door. Katie knew she needed a better solution, yet she didn't want to admit the inevitable truth that Trixie was suffering.

It was Saturday and after she had dropped Joan home and was running a bath for Lucy, Jack came in with a very self-satisfied look on his face.

"I've got a surprise for you. Come and see."

"Oh, how lovely. Do I need to come now."

The exaggerated sigh and the pointed look suggested she did. She turned off the taps, checked the girls were happy watching TV and followed Jack outside. He led her to the garage. To her amazement when she went inside it was transformed. There was a partition across the back third and a small staircase leading upwards where a ladder used to be. The room above had been used to store things they hadn't been ready to part with: the old pram and cot, outgrown toys and old vinyl recordings that they could no longer play, which were too much part of their youth to part with. Then there was furniture that had no place in this house, that they had liked in their previous homes. In other words, it was a junk room. As Katie climbed the stairs her eyes grew wider. The walls were painted pristine white with photo tiles progressing upwards: pictures of the children or pretty views. She paused to stare at one of them and tugged Jack's sleeve.

"Where did you get these?"

"One of those deals where you get a free one every month. Just pay postage."

"But the pictures. Where…"

"Off your phone when you weren't looking." He grinned. "Come on you've not seen anything yet."

Shaking her head in wonderment, Katie followed him to the top of the stairs where there was a tiny landing. Two doors opened off it. Jack opened one to show the prettiest little cloakroom with a sparkling new toilet and tiny corner basin. The walls were pink and there was a pot of artificial flowers on the sill of the narrow, slit window.

Bewildered Katie watched as he opened the second door. This time she gasped. The room was painted a bright sunny yellow. A single bed with a pretty flower decked duvet took up most of the space and a thin chest of drawers stood in the corner. A little bedside table was squeezed by the bed with a lamp on top. More photos adorned the walls.

"Don't worry about the old junk. I created a storage space under the rafters, it's all there. Well, most of it anyway and what isn't needed to go."

Katie gazed round the room trying to take the change in. Why, why on earth…

"It's only for weekends mind you."

"Huh?"

"Katie have you even been listening."

"Sorry I am just stunned. You did all this?"

"Well not exactly. I had a plumber do the loo of course and a carpenter fixed up the floor. I did the painting. Your friend from that course you went to helped me choose the décor. The photos were her idea."

"But why? What is it for?"

It was Jack's turn to look bewildered. "Really? You can't guess?"

Katie shook her head.

"It's for your mother of course. She can sleep here at the weekends. Then we don't need to traipse back and forth so much. I've even set up a baby monitor so you can hear her if she gets up in the night and wanders off."

"What about Trixie?"

"Seriously I do all this and all you can say is what about that blasted dog!"

"I can't leave her at Mum's alone all weekend."

"Honestly Katie you are the limit! I worked so hard on this to make our lives a bit easier and all you can do is hone in on the one flaw in my plan! Can't you just be grateful!"

Katie realised her mistake and pushing Trixie aside as the problem to be solved later, she threw her arms around her husband.

"Thank you sweetheart, it is lovely. Mum will love it. It is amazing."

Mollified Jack smiled.

Katie took one last glance around, she wasn't ungrateful, it was beautiful. However, Jack didn't know her mother so well as she did. She knew Joan would struggle up the narrow stairs. She would find the toilet too small and having to leave the little bedroom and then open another door to reach it would confuse her. Joan's disorientation would mean she would struggle with the sloped ceiling. It was a lovely idea and for a while it might work. How she wished Jack had run the idea past her first.

And what about the poor dog?

Chapter 41

Bonfire Night

November 2019

Katie was beginning to relax. She had her job under control and her arrangements for her mum were working reasonably well. Of course, there were random days like the one when her mother had inexplicably decided she was a ballroom dancer and insisted Katie practiced with her. There were still the strange notes that kept popping up with instructions or memos that her mother would tell her "Katy had written," when Katie knew she hadn't. However, on a day-to-day basis it all seemed to be OK. Or was she kidding herself? Jack had solved the weekend problems most of the time by building that room. Her mother had been enchanted by it and as long as Katie escorted her upstairs to bed and then dashed up first thing in the morning, Joan was coping with the tiny cloakroom. There had been a couple of night-time accidents, when Katie had quietly washed the bedding and popped her mother discretely in the family bath in the morning.

She had solved the problem of Trixie, at least for now. She had found a dog sitter who would take her for the weekends. It cost Katie £40 a week which she paid in cash so Jack would not know. It felt deceitful, although Katie reasoned that she had earned the money so she could spend it. She knew Jack would eventually notice the increased cash withdrawals. However, for now it was working. Trixie looked healthier and happier as she was properly fed, walked and groomed at the weekends at least.

It felt like life might go smoothly for a little while after all.

Lucy was excited. Bonfire Night was coming. She absolutely adored Bonfire Night. Matt's school hosted a fabulous evening every year. She loved standing by the massive hot fire that had taken days to build, feeling its warmth. She could see the framework was ready when they went past Matt's school. It wouldn't be long now, just 5 more sleeps! There was a smaller fire too, where supervised children could toast marshmallows. Daddy always helped her with that, a small, significant moment of connection to her father. Best of all were the fireworks. Daddy would lift her on his shoulders where she could see above the crowd. The sky blazed with sparkling colours accompanied by loud bangs, whooshes and fizzes. Molly would stand close to Mummy and cover her ears, but Lucy loved the noise and the flashing colours. It was amazing and she simply couldn't wait!

She was daydreaming about it when she heard her parents arguing. They were quarrelling about Bonfire Night!

"Really Katie can't we have one night out as a family without your mother!"

"It is a Friday night and I always bring Mum here on Fridays."

"Yes, about that. We are going to have to miss a weekend soon so we can visit my parents."

"Oh, can't you just go with the children?"

"No, not again, mother feels like you are avoiding her. We did agree you would come."

"Surely you have explained I can't leave Mum alone."

"You do on your workdays."

"Yes, but I make arrangements on those days!"

"Then make arrangements on a weekend. We are going to see my parents on the first weekend in December. They are going on a Christmas cruise this year, so they want to see us all before they go."

Lucy shrank back from the tone of Daddy's voice. He was getting cross. She didn't like it when he was cross. Maybe she could fix things. Not about the weekend at Grandpa and Nanny's but maybe about Bonfire Night. She bounced into the room.

"Mummy, Daddy I have an idea!"

Both parents paused and turned to look at their daughter. Katie silently hoping she hadn't heard the raised voices.

"Yes sweetheart, what is it?"

"It's about Bonfire Night. Can Grandma come too? She can hold Molly's hand when she is scared and then you can enjoy the fireworks more Mummy. You still have to lift me up though Daddy."

Jack sighed. Katie realised Lucy had heard and while that concerned her, she was secretly glad of her little daughter's intervention. She turned to Jack.

"What do you think?"

"I can't fight you both, so yes, I suppose Grandma can come. We are still going to my parents though, so make those arrangements." He stomped off back to his newspaper.

Katie looked down at Lucy. "Thank you sweetheart, I know Bonfire Night is your special night. It is kind of you to want to share it with Grandma."

Lucy beamed. "She's going to love it!"

Joan was confused. Katie had been so rushed when she had come to collect her, bundling poor Trixie into the car. What on earth had she done with the dog? They had left her somewhere. She missed her dog, but she did like going to Katie's. However, they weren't there. They were outside in a cold field and Lucy was crying.

"We are late Mummy, we are too far back, I can't feel the fire and we didn't see them light it! And I won't see the fireworks from here!"

"Of course, you will, Daddy will pick you up."

"But Daddy isn't here!"

"He will be soon."

"But he isn't now!"

"Then I will pick you up."

"You can't put me on your shoulders!"

"You are right Squirt, Mum can't but I can!" Matt interjected. For once he hadn't run off with his mates and was with the family, hovering near the gate. Katie had planned to pick up her mother and join them there, while Jack took the children. However, Jack had inevitably got stuck in a last-minute meeting and she had had to bundle them all over to get Joan. The traffic had been awful, and they were late. Jack had asked them to meet him at the gate, as in the dark they would never find each other in the huge crowd on the massive field. However, the bonfire had been lit and Lucy had missed it. They mustn't miss the fireworks.

"Right," said Katie, whipping out her phone. I'm going to tell Dad we have gone on in. Hopefully he will find us but there's no point us hanging around here and missing out. Come on Lucy dry your eyes, Matt will lift you up."

She pinged a text to Jack, knowing he wouldn't read it until he arrived as he was driving, so he couldn't object and took hold of Lucy's hand. Joan hovered back.

"Let's go Mum," she said, reaching back with her other hand. "Come with us."

"I think I will just go home dear, it's a bit cold for me out here."

"It will be warm by the fire come on."

Reluctantly Joan followed.

Matt was as good as his word and hoisted Lucy up onto his shoulders. Katie marvelled at how much he had grown while she wasn't watching. She thought wistfully of those early days when he was the one Jack was swinging in the air. Where was Jack?

Joan was getting colder. Her feet were frozen. Katie had made her wear wellies as the field was muddy. They were old and leaked and her feet were wet. She had two jumpers on under her coat yet still she shivered. Her gloves were wet too from leaning on a post to steady herself when they went through the gate. Her fingers felt stiff and hurt.

Then the noises began. The first bang startled her and she looked around to see if anyone was hurt. Molly looked alarmed as she had her hands over her ears. Lucy was laughing, balanced up there on Matt's shoulders. That didn't look safe. Joan took a step backwards. Another bang! Then a whooshing sound and red flashes in the sky. Something was wrong. She remembered those noises.

More bangs, fizzes and shrieks from the people around her.

She remembered! You needed to get to a shelter. Mummy would take her. She looked around. Where were her parents. Why was everyone outside? It was a raid! They needed to run to somewhere safe!

Her mind raced as the flashes continued. Where on earth was she and what should she do?

She stepped back again, her ears hurt from the noise. She stood on the foot of the man behind her. He yelled at her to "watch out!" and she mumbled an apology.

Another huge bang and her mind cleared. She must go to the shelter on Beech Avenue. Mummy had always said if she was ever caught in a raid she should go there. Mummy also said she should ask for help if she needed it. She looked around her. No one else was moving. Who could she ask? No, she must be brave and go alone. She turned and walked as swiftly as she could away from the flashing bombs and into the dark.

The fireworks ended. Katie had loved watching her children. Molly had been fearful of the noise as usual but had enjoyed the colours. Lucy and Matt had connected better than she had ever remembered. And what a display it had been. Poor Jack had missed out. Maybe he was in the field somewhere. She supposed she had better look for him. Or at least check her phone.

"Mummy, can Matt and I get marshmallows?"

"I'm afraid you need an adult for that and Matt is not quite that yet; although he did a great job holding you up. Let me just see if Dad has arrived and then we will all go. Grandma likes marshmallows too don't you Mum? Mum?"

The mass of people had homogenised into a large blob. Her mother must be nearby. She squinted to try to make her out."

"Use your phone torch Mum," suggested Matt."

"I can't see Grandma. Did you see where she went? She was right next to me!" She swept the torch over the field. No sign of her mother. Not again!

"We need to find her. She must be here somewhere."

"But the marshmallows will all be gone!"

"I'm sorry Lucy we have to find her first. She can't be far."

Lucy screwed up her face and folded her arms. This was her night and it was all going so horribly wrong. Mummy didn't care, she just grabbed her arm and practically dragged her across the field. Matt and Molly followed.

"Maybe she went towards the gate. There's only one way out and they close it during the show. If we hurry, they won't have opened it yet for people to leave." shouted Matt above the din.

He was probably right. It was such a big field and Joan probably wouldn't even find the gate.

Suddenly the loudspeaker boomed.

"We have an elderly lady here who is a bit confused. If anyone has lost a grandma, please come to the refreshment tent." Sighing with relief Katie headed that way. Sure enough she found Joan standing arguing with Mr Tucker, a teacher from Matt's school.

"We need to get to the shelter. It isn't safe out here. Mummy always told me I must go there. Which way is it?"

"What are you talking about Mum?"

Joan's bewildered face seemed momentarily to not recognise her own daughter. Then it cleared and she smiled.

"Katie! You know where the shelter is don't you?"

"It seems your mother has had a bit of a memory lapse. I think she thinks there's an air raid. Someone found her wandering around looking for the shelter and brought her to me. I imagine the noise of the fireworks triggered it."

"What? But Mum it is 2019. The war was over 74 years ago! When you were 10!"

"I don't understand. Where's Mummy?"

Joan stood there shivering and frightened. Whatever had happened in her mind had obviously terrified her.

"Let's just get you home and warmed up Mum."

"But Mummy! I want my marshmallows!"

"Don't be silly Lucy, Grandma needs to go home. Marshmallows aren't important." Her own shock and delayed panic sharpened Katie's response.

Lucy burst into tears. "It's not fair, today was my favourite. Daddy didn't come and now Grandma has ruined it."

Mr Tucker had been turning back to his duties but at Lucy's outburst he turned back.

"Is that your little sister Matthew?"

"Yes sir."

"If you hang on just a minute, I will find a bag of marshmallows you can take with you. Might cheer her up a bit."

"Thank you sir."

Mr Tucker did as promised and shamed by his kindness, Katie softened her tone.

"Come on Lucy, let's go home. Daddy is there waiting for us as he was too late to come at all. I will ask him to make your own little bonfire in the garden and the three of you can toast your treats. OK?"

Katie linked one arm through her mother's and held Lucy's hand with the other. Lucy clutched her sweets to her chest and stumbled along beside her. She didn't know why Mummy was angry. She was frightened by Grandma's odd behaviour and her big night had been spoiled. Tears tricked down her face and she noticed Molly was crying too. Matt saw them both and put an arm around each of them.

"C'mon you two. I'll help you toast the mallows. Biggest one for me though!" He grinned. Lucy sniffed. Matt was never this nice to her. The whole day was just weird.

Chapter 42

Baking

November 2019

"Oh how lovely! A cake sale!" Joan looked at the leaflet that had been thrust through her door:

Cake sale

Methodist Church

10.00

Sat 23rd November

Donations of baked goods welcome

She stared at it, slowly digesting its contents. Saturday, hmm, it wasn't Saturday today. She knew that as the bin men had just been and they didn't come on Saturdays. So she had a few days. She could make cakes! What fun! She went to her kitchen. What ingredients would she need? What sort of cakes would she make? She thought carefully.

"Chocolate!" she said out loud, "I like chocolate cake best!"

She started opening cupboards. She found a cake tin, a bowl and a big wooden spoon. Then she searched for ingredients. She had flour and sugar but no chocolate powder. She thought hard. She would need eggs too. And something else from the fridge. She shook her head. It wouldn't come. Never mind she would go to the shops to get the chocolate powder and ask them.

She pulled on her coat and shoes. She took the key from the hook by the door, prompted by Katie's prominent notice and smiling to herself she set off to the shops.

"I'm going to make a chocolate cake," she announced at the till. The young woman stared at her. There was a queue, the old lady had no shopping.

"I need ingredients?"

The girl shrugged, "You'll find them on the shelves."

Joan hesitated, "Yes but I'm not sure what I need?"

The girl just stared at her while the man in the queue behind shuffled uncomfortably.

"Can you help me?" asked Joan smiling hopefully.

"I have to help this queue first," muttered the girl.

"Oh yes of course, I'll wait then," stuttered Joan.

The queue kept growing while Joan stood and watched. The girl studiously avoided her eyes. Half an hour passed.

"Excuse me love can I help you?" a warm smile turned on Joan. Sally, a mother of three started work at the tills later in the morning after her school run. "You just look a bit lost there."

"Oh yes thank you. There was something I needed." Joan screwed up her face in concentration.

"Chocolate cake." Muttered the girl.

"Oh, we have lots of lovely cakes to choose from, follow me."

Two minutes later Joan left the shop clutching a large, beautifully iced cake.

As she walked into her kitchen to put it away, she noticed all the baking things out on the counter. She looked at the cake in her hand. She shook her head. She had got it wrong again, hadn't she?

She caught sight of the leaflet. She picked it up. Oh yes, she was going to bake! She looked around. She had everything she needed. Except…

"Butter!" she exclaimed, "I need butter!"

She looked in the fridge. Next to the butter was a large lemon. I can make a lemon cake she thought. Excellent.

She picked up the butter and put it in the bowl. She frowned. What was next. She shook her head slowly trying to remember.

She poured in the flour.

She cracked each egg from her fridge carefully and added them one by one. Six in total.

She added a whole bag of sugar.

She forgot the lemon.

She picked up her spoon and started to stir. The butter was hard, straight from the fridge and wouldn't blend in with the rest. The eggs, flour and sugar made a gloopy mess. She stared at her bowl. Something was wrong. She looked around the kitchen. In the corner was a gleaming mixer. Katie had given it to her years ago for Christmas. She had carefully unpacked it and plugged it in telling Joan how much time it would save her. Joan had smiled gratefully but she had preferred to cook the traditional way, so the mixer remained untouched.

However, now she seized on it. She carefully poured her mixture into the bowl. She pressed the start button. The machine burst into life. Joan jumped back at the noise. The beaters churned and spat, breaking the lumpy butter into smaller and smaller pieces. The eggs grew frothy on the top. Then finally, miraculously it all homogenised into a smooth mass. She pressed stop.

Smiling she poured it carefully into her cake tin. She put it in the oven.

Then she went into the living room to wait.

A loud buzzing woke Joan with a start! Someone was at the door. There was a smell coming from the kitchen, rather a nice smell. She went to open the door. It was Katie!

"Hello Mum just thought I'd pop in to make you some lunch." Katie smiled brightly.

"How lovely," replied Joan. Come on in!

"What's that smell?" Katie rushed into the kitchen and opened the oven. There, inexplicably, was a cake, perfectly risen but slightly singed at the edges. She looked around for oven gloves and carefully lifted it out.

"Whatever made you make that Mum?" worry creased her face. "You haven't used the oven for ages.

"I felt like making a cake I suppose," said Joan. She crossed her arms and starred at Katie, reminding her of Lucy when she had been caught out misbehaving.

"Well I got here just in time to get it out of the oven, didn't I? Maybe next time you should set the timer to remind you when it is cooked?" The thought of her mother baking regularly scared her but what if she put a note on the oven about setting the timer? It had worked with the kettle and toaster. She shook her head willing the frightening thoughts of fire engines' sirens screeching out of her head.

"Oh I probably won't make another one for ages," said Joan airily. "Now shall we have a slice?"

Katie tried to release the hot cake from its tin, but it was firmly stuck. Clearly Joan had forgotten to grease or line the ancient tin and its non-stick properties were long gone. She fished around in the cutlery drawer to find a palate knife. She slid it around the sides loosening the cake as much as possible. Eventually it flopped out, leaving much of the base stuck to the tin. Using the knife Katie deftly scrapped the last piece out and pressed it onto the bottom of the upside down cake.

"There, let's let it cool just a little and with luck it will all stick together. In the meantime, let's tidy up a bit."

Ten minutes later the kitchen gleamed, the kettle was boiled and Katie sat down with her mother to eat the sweetest slice of sponge cake she had ever tasted!

Chapter 43

Cake Sale

December 2019

Joan wasn't quite sure what she was supposed to do today. She had checked the calendar but as she had no idea what day it was how could she know? She rummaged in the kitchen pile of papers to see if there were any clues. There was a leaflet- a cake sale! Something stirred in her memory. Hadn't she made a cake for this? She looked in the cupboard. There in a tin at the back was a beautifully iced chocolate cake. She stared at it, admiring her handiwork. Then gently lifted it out and searching again found a ribbon to tie around it.

"Perfect!" she exclaimed.

From the leaflet Joan ascertained that the cake sale was at the Church Hall. At 10.00am. She looked at her clock. It said 9.30 so she had plenty of time. Carefully she put the cake, resplendent with its ribbon back into the cake tin. She found her coat and shoes and stuffing the leaflet into her pocket she set off.

It was a long walk to the C of E Church, left at the end of the lane and a way down the hill. She was tired when she got there. The door to the hall was firmly locked. She looked around. No sign of anyone. How odd. It must be nearly 10.00 by now. She stood, tapping her feet impatiently. The air was cold, it was early December. Not that Joan realised that. Her breath froze and her fingers holding the tin started to get numb.

"Excuse me?" A man was smiling at her. "Can I help you? You look a little lost."

"Well, um I…"

"What have you got there?" he said gently.

"Oh yes!" said Joan brightly. "A cake for the sale!"

The vicar frowned for a second and then mustered his best smile.

"Well, you are a little, um, early- it isn't till...um...tomorrow!"

"Oh dear," said Joan.

"But don't worry, why don't you leave the cake with me? I will make sure it's put into the sale in the morning. Save you coming back again."

"Oh yes that would be lovely- thank you!"

"No problem. It's very kind of you to bake for us."

"I enjoyed it!" said Joan, handing over her tin and beaming with pleasure. She turned to go.

"Are you alright to walk home alone?" asked the man.

"Oh yes I got here, didn't I?" laughed Joan.

"Well thank you again. Goodbye."

"Goodbye!"

The vicar took the cake into the hall to set up for his parochial meeting. They could put it to good use as refreshments he supposed. They hadn't had a cake sale for months. The only one he had heard of was weeks ago at the Methodists. Poor old thing probably had dementia like so many of his parishioners. No one young ever seemed to come to Church anymore. At least not to his. He was swamped with elderly ladies like that one who needed more care and support than he could provide. Families didn't seem to have time to care for their old folks anymore. He hoped she would find her way home alright. She wasn't one of his and he really had enough of his own to worry about. He set the cake in the middle of the table and pulled out his notes ready for the members to arrive, brushing the old lady from his thoughts.

Joan was so cold. Her fingers hurt. She had walked up the hill and turned left but somehow her house didn't seem to be where she had left it. Her toes were starting to freeze too now as she stumbled on. She was heading into the woods. That wasn't right. The woods were the other end of the lane. Not where her house was. Confused she turned around. The wind whipped her head and she wished she was home in the warm. Whatever made her go out on a day like this? Scared now she looked frantically around for help. No sign of anyone but there was some traffic back the way she had come. She walked on. If she could stop a car, she could get some help. She started waving at the cars, but no one stopped. A little child waved back and a few people smiled at the old lady waving at them. She was cold and tired and lost and couldn't think what to do. Just keep walking she told herself. You will get there eventually. She didn't see the ice, her frozen feet skidded back and she fell forward. A sharp pain shot through her knee and with her hands too slow to protect her, her face bashed hard on the solid icy ground.

The vicar took one bite of the stale co-op cake.
"Um…probably best not to eat this…one of the older members of my flock…think it's about as old as her…

"Mrs Robinson, Mrs Thomas would like to see you."
"OK I'll pop into her office at break time."
"Er no she wants to see you now."
It was only 9.30, she'd only just started her maths lesson. What on earth…but the secretary's fixed smile and anxious look rang alarm bells in Katie's head.
"Um OK- who will take over here?"
"I'm to watch them for a few minutes till another teacher arrives."
Panic coursed through Katie. Something was seriously wrong. What had she done? A thousand scenarios ran through her mind. Had someone complained? Perhaps a parent? A child? A colleague? She couldn't think of a mistake she could have made to be pulled out of class mid-lesson by the Head and replaced by the secretary. Mustering her firmest teacher voice, she asked the children to put down their pencils and fetch their reading books. It would be easier for Miss Clarke to manage some silent reading.

Miss Clarke looked increasingly anxious as Katie told the children she wouldn't be long and they were to sit quietly with their books till she got back. The sympathetic smile she shot Katie as she left did nothing to calm her panic. She was beginning to think she was about to be fired. But why?

"Do take a seat Katie." Mrs Thomas had the same gentle trying-to-be-kind look as Miss Clarke. With a jolt, her fear for her job was replaced by terror for her children. Had there been an accident?

"We have just had a call from the hospital…"

"Which one?" whispered Katie.

"Oh, St Barts"

"No… I mean which of my children."

"It's not your children Katie. We believe it is your mother. Is her name Joan?"

Relief and new worry fuzzed Katie's head.

"Yes, yes Joan Jessup. What has happened to her?"

"When did you last see or speak to her?"

Guilt replaced fear as Katie realised she hadn't actually managed to get hold of Joan over the weekend. At least not since early Saturday. Jack had insisted she go with him to his parents for the weekend and despite numerous attempts to check on her mother Joan hadn't picked up the phone. She had put it down to her mother's new habit of leaving the phone off the hook, which meant the handset didn't charge. Jack had objected to her rushing over there when they got back, saying it would spoil a nice weekend. Instead, she had been planning to pop round there after work, before she collected the children from after school club.

"Saturday morning."

"Well on Saturday evening an elderly lady was found unconscious lying in the snow on St Catherine's Hill by two passers-by. She was taken to hospital by ambulance. She had no ID on her. Once she was stable, she said her name was Joan, but didn't seem to have any other memory of who she was or where she belonged. As nobody came looking for her over the weekend the hospital has been ringing round GP surgeries in the area this morning to find anyone who meets her description and suffers from dementia. They may have other leads too, but they think it could be your mother. They have been ringing your mobile which obviously you haven't answered as you were teaching. They had the school's number too, so they rang here."

"Oh… I had better go to the hospital…is that OK? Do you have cover for my class? My planning is all on the server."

"Of course. While Miss Clarke fetched you, I rang the supply agency and help is on its way. But that is not your problem. We need to get you to the hospital to see if it is indeed your mother and find out how she is."

"Thank you," stuttered Katie, "I need to collect my bag from class. My car keys are in it."

"I'll go, you sit there, you have had a shock and I don't think you would want your class to see you looking so white. You won't be needing your car keys. I shall be driving you. It isn't wise to drive when so worried. Besides then you can try ringing your mother again just in case she is safely at home." With that she swept out of the room leaving Katie to try to rearrange her thoughts into some coherent pattern.

The receptionist at the hospital took an age locating "Joan". Mrs Thomas had carefully explained the circumstances and eventually she was found to be in the acute admissions unit. There the receptionist was less friendly, almost hostile.

"The lady you are looking for is in bay 4. There's a member of the adult social care team with her now. If it your mother, she will want to know what's going on with her care."

"Thank you but right now I am sure you would like us to identify the lady wouldn't you. Then, if it is Mrs Jessup, we will need to see her doctor. Can you arrange that please?"

Kate silently thanked heaven Mrs Thomas was there to take charge.

"Of course. Just come back to me." The receptionist was cowed a little by the headmistress's tone.

Katie stepped towards the bed. There, shrunken against the stark white mattress was her mother with a large bruise across her forehead.

"Oh Mum, whatever have you done!" Tears coursed Katie's cheeks as she took hold of her mother's hand, completely ignoring the woman by the bed.

"Katie dear?"

"Yes Mum, it's me. I'm here. It's all going to be alright."

"I'll fetch the doctor." said Mrs Thomas.

Overall, the doctor explained, Joan had been lucky. She had dislocated her knee when she fell. They had slipped it back into place relatively easily and with care and rest it should resolve itself. She was suffering from hyperthermia when she came in, but thankfully some people had found her before nightfall. Though they estimated she had lain there for several hours.

He followed this with a stream of information and questions regarding Joan's state of mind and lack of care. Katie tried to absorb his words while stroking Joan's hand and blinking back her tears. His biggest concern was her level of confusion. Did she have a dementia diagnosis? And if so, why was she wandering around alone? The duty social worker was with her now. It would depend on her finances if she qualified for any level of state care, although it was obvious she needed something. Physically she should fully recover from her ordeal, although it may trigger a downward spiral with her dementia. No one knew why that happened, but it was fairly predictable that it would. Now she was identified unfortunately they really needed to clear the bed. They would hold off as long as they could while Katie talked things through with the duty social worker. In the end Katie just nodded. She had tried to explain she had only been gone for the weekend. He wasn't interested. He had done his bit so now it was over to the social worker.

She sat, pencil at the ready staring at Katie. Another stream of questions and information poured from her lips.

"So, can Joan be safely released into your care? What are her living arrangements? She isn't on our list, so does she have a private care package, or do you manage alone? We can't offer a huge amount of support. We are very over stretched but if she qualifies for help, we can do a six-week assessment."

"Um so far, I take care of her. She lives alone, just with her dog. Trixie! Oh no poor Trixie! Was she with her when she fell or is she shut up at home?"

"I know nothing about a dog."

"Look, "said Mrs Thomas, taking charge once more. I really ought to be heading back to school and clearly you two have much to discuss, although it can probably wait, as I'm sure Katie would rather spend some time reassuring her mother."

Joan, a benign smile on her face, had dropped off to sleep once she had felt Katie's hand in hers.

The social worker nodded and handed a card to Katie.

"I will be in touch later today. We must speak before your mother leaves the hospital and she cannot go home alone."

"Of course she won't! She will stay with me."

With a nod to Mrs Thomas and a last glance at Joan, the social worker left.

"Obviously, Katie you need to take some time to sort out your mother's needs, so I won't expect you in school this week. Take your time and get help where it is available. I will ask Miss Clarke to contact your husband and tell him where you are. He can collect your car from school and the children if need be."

Katie smiled inwardly, conceding that Miss Clarke and Mrs Thomas probably would achieve the impossible and get Jack to manage childcare.

"As for the dog, if you like I can pop into your mother's house on the way to check if it is there. If it's not I will have Miss Clarke ring around the local shelters. I'm sure the dog can be found. I will need a key of course."

"I don't know how to thank you, for everything," Katie rummaged in her bag, scribbled her mother's address on a piece of paper and found the door key.

Mrs Thomas smiled wistfully. "My mother had dementia."

Chapter 44

Social Worker

December 2019

"What are you going to do for your mother?"

Katie blinked at the social worker. What kind of a question was that? Her mother had been staying with her since her accident. As her knee had made climbing up to her special room impossible, she had been sleeping in the children's playroom. They had been very good about moving out their toys and playing upstairs, although the big sticking point had been the television. Katie had never allowed televisions in their rooms but having to share the main living room one between them all had been a nightmare.

Lucy had often snuck in with Grandma, who was happy to watch cartoons if it meant she could cuddle her granddaughter. Molly just quietly accepted the situation. However, Jack and Matt had clashed horribly over how much football was to be watched in a week. Katie had not returned to work since her mother's fall. There had only been a couple of weeks of term left and then it had been Christmas holidays. She knew she had to go back for the new term. And quite honestly it was a strain having her mother there all the time. Especially on Jack who found the endless repeats of the same questions or stories exhausting.

However social services had been monitoring Joan ever since she left the hospital and were now insisting on a 'care package' if she was to return to her house.

The social worker sat tall and upright in Katie's kitchen. Her nose was slightly hooked, which made Katie feel like she was being watched over by an imperious eagle waiting to swoop and carry her away to her lair.

She blinked again and answered carefully.

"Before Mum's accident she spent most weekends with us. I visited every day I wasn't working and made sure she had meals prepared. I had her shopping delivered and she has a cleaner. On the days I do work she had an activity to go to each day or the day centre to attend. She never spent the whole day alone if I could avoid it."

"Yes, that's all well and good but she still managed to wander off and have a serious accident. We are trying to avoid a repeat."

"I appreciate that but…"

"So," the social worker cut her off. "I will assume that she is living alone and will need a full package. That is 4 visits per day. One to get her up, one for lunch, one for dinner and a bedtime check to get her to bed. Does she need help in the shower?"

"She has a bath."

"That won't do. Far too long. We will have to do a sitting wash. Perhaps you can help her bathe when you visit."

"The bath runs quite quickly, she just loves to have a soak, she never liked showers."

"Visits are 15 minutes, there simply isn't time. A shower is much more practical. I would suggest fitting one, but I appreciate your mother has no funds."

Katie smarted inwardly and almost offered to pay for it herself. Then remembering her mother's preference, she held back. She would help her mum bathe when she could.

"NRS healthcare will do a house assessment and fit some equipment. They can put in rails for her to hold in the bathroom and a special toilet seat. They can also put flood monitors in case she leaves the taps running. There are various bits of kitchen equipment too. And an alarm on the door that will sound if she tries to leave alone. You will have to show any visitors how to turn it off. And a key safe for carers to get in. If she has medication, which I assume she does, there is a medication pot that buzzes to tell her to take them and has daily slots. You will have to fill it and monitor. Our carers can't dispense medication. You will need to provide meals too. It is best to have those delivered. The microwavable ones. There's no time for much else. Sandwich ingredients are useful too."

"Hold on, what if Mum wants to pop to the local shop or take her dog for a walk. She needs to know how to go out and not set off an alarm."

The eagle looked down her imperious nose at Katie.

"I think the days of walking alone are over. The dog is a trip hazard too. I don't think your mother is capable of caring for it either. Best you keep it here."

Katie winced. Trixie had been thriving in the dog sitters where she had been for almost a month now. Jack had never asked about her and Katie had quietly paid the bills. Even she could see that time was up.

"She isn't here. My husband is allergic. She is being looked after for now."

"Well make that permanent. Your mother has probably forgotten she ever had a dog."

Katie looked down to hide the welling tears. She had battled so hard and for so long. Now this wretched woman was taking over. This was her mother, her choices, not some social worker's. And poor Molly. She loved that dog. Katie bit her lip.

The woman softened. "I know none of this is easy. Dementia is cruel. We do what we can, but reality is your mother would probably be safest in a care home."

"She doesn't want to. And we can't afford one anyway unless we sell her house and that would take time."

"There are state run ones, she would qualify. I'm aware there are no places available locally. I could look further afield or put her on the waiting list."

Katie shook her head. "No let's try this first."

It was all soon settled. Joan would move back into her home two days before Katie returned to school. NRS would visit and assess first, then return and fit all the gadgets and alarms she needed. Then the carers would start their pattern of daily visits. Everything else would continue as before. Katie hoped it would make her feel that her mother was safe. Yet she wasn't sure. She needed a sympathetic voice to chat to. As soon as the social worker left, she phoned Maddy.

After outlining the details, she asked her opinion.

"It sounds as good as you will get. But don't be surprised if not all the visits happen."

"What do you mean?"

"Carers are poorly paid and over worked. If there is a crisis at one place they stay and sort that first. They have their own illnesses and family issues to deal with. I'm not saying they are bad, just there aren't enough of them and if there is anything out of the ordinary it all falls apart. And obviously with dementia there is often something out of the ordinary."

"How do you know all this. You don't use them."

"No, I did for a bit when I wanted to still work. But it wasn't OK, so I quit. And did it myself."

"I didn't know that."

"I don't talk about it much. It's all long ago."

"Do you think I should quit my job?"

"Your situation is so different to mine. You have children and it's your mother not your husband. You have a whole world of spinning plates. I can't advise you on those."

Katie sighed. "I just don't know what to do. I think we should try this first. It might be OK."

"It might. But one thing you must do is rehome that poor dog."

"I know. I have known that for ages. Molly will be devastated."

"When did Molly last see the dog?"

"To be honest it was before the accident."

"So do it quietly and tell her later. And meantime get her a pet of her own."

"I can't. Jack's allergic."

"Only to fur! Get her a tortoise, a lizard, or a fish! Or even a snake!" Maddy laughed. "But whatever you do make sure she takes care of it herself. You have enough plates to spin!"

Chapter 45

Goodbye Trixie

December 2019

In the end, after all her agonising, the Trixie problem resolved itself. Katie had popped over to the dog sitters to pay the latest bill. It was 22nd December and she was greeted by a smiling sitter and an excited dog. As she sat on the sofa with Trixie curled on her lap the sitter took a visible breath and then began.

"I thought it was time we had a chat. Now it isn't that I don't like taking care of Trixie and you have certainly paid me well for it. However, I have always promised my husband I wouldn't have dogs in over Christmas. Now don't panic we are all willing to make an exception for this little one. Although now, with her best interests at heart, I think we need to look at a more permanent solution. I have another client, well two actually, a lovely couple. They have always had dogs, little fluffy ones like Trixie. Their last one died just over a month ago. They are utterly bereft but don't feel able to start over with a puppy. They are both in their 70's but very fit and well. I wondered, well, how would you feel about them taking on Trixie? I know your mother loves her, yet from what you have told me and quite frankly from the state she was in when I first had her, I don't think it right to send her back. I know your daughter loves her and the couple have said she can visit any time she likes. I would have her here every other weekend like I did their previous dog, as they go to stay with their daughter who doesn't allow dogs on her cream carpets. So Trixie would have some familiar faces in her life still."

She finally paused for another breath, "Sorry that all came out in a rush, I've been rehearsing all day!"

"Yes please," whispered Katie as tears rolled down her cheeks, "Oh yes please."

Katie decided to take Molly with her to hand over Trixie the very next day. The Carters lived in a neat little semi just two roads down from the sitter's house. She had offered to do the exchange at her house, but Katie wanted to see where Trixie would be living. Katie rang the doorbell and was greeted almost instantly by an upright gentleman with grey whiskers and a neat comb over. His wife was short and plump with sparkling blue eyes.

"Oh hello sweetheart!" the wife exclaimed, ignoring Katie and reaching out towards Trixie. "Aren't you just adorable!"

"Sorry," muttered the husband, "She's been so excited all morning, like a child expecting her first puppy! Do come in."

Katie entered with Molly clutching her hand tightly.

Mrs Carter lifted her head from petting Trixie and beamed at Molly.

"So, you must be Molly," she said gently, "I believe you have been responsible for keeping this little dog happy while your grandma has been poorly. And that you would like to visit her sometimes? I would love that. You can take her in the garden to play ball now if you like?"

Molly nodded mutely and Mr Carter showed her out into the back garden. There was a selection of balls waiting ready for Trixie and Molly was soon engrossed in play.

Katie accepted a cup of tea and sat down in the kitchen.

"We appreciate how hard this must be for you." said Mrs Carter. I can't imagine having to part with such a dear little dog. I promise you she will be loved and cherished if you are happy for us to have her." A small crease appeared in her forehead, "Are you happy? Do you need to know anything more about us? Trixie would have two walks a day, good quality food and a regular brush. I always did our dear Roxy on a Friday evening. Found it very soothing. Then more often in the winter when she got muddy- those types of coats need lots of care, so they don't get matted. I believe you know we go away every other weekend and she would go to the sitters, but of course- that's how you found us."

Katie smiled and quickly soothed away the older woman's worry.

"I am thrilled Trixie is to have such a happy new home. I would keep her myself, but my husband is allergic. My only concern is Molly. Would you really be happy for her to visit? It would probably only be at weekends. Would that be an intrusion?"

"We would love to see her, don't worry about that. Poor child it must be so hard for her. Why don't we say you will come every other weekend- the ones we are here. And maybe more often in the holidays? I will give you my number and you can give me a ring to check we are in. The only regular time we wouldn't be is Sunday evening as we go to evensong at our local Church. Obviously, we pop out to the shops and would be going for walks. So best ring first as I don't want you to waste a journey." The old lady bustled about finding pen and paper and writing down a landline number.

She smiled as she handed it over, "We did try a mobile but kept forgetting to charge it. And they are so intrusive, they keep going off in the shops and on walks. There's an answer machine if you miss us and we always check it don't we love?"

Her husband nodded and smiled, clearly happy for his wife to do the talking.

"Shall we bring Molly and Trixie in now?" suggested Mrs Carter. "I can show her where Trixie will sleep and be fed, so she is sure she will have all she needs."

Katie nodded and watched as the gentle, older lady helped her daughter see just how loved the little dog would be, as she took her all over the house with Trixie trotting behind sniffing excitedly at everything.

"So Molly, do you think Trixie will be happy here?"

Katie watched anxiously as her daughter nodded and gave a little smile.

"Good, I am so glad you approve. Now I have spoken to your mum about you visiting. She has my number and you are both welcome as often as we can all manage. And if you just want to ring and check Trixie is OK that's fine too. It will be important to her that she still sees you sometimes. Clearly, she loves you very much."

As if on cue the little dog reached up and licked Molly's hand. Katie saw Molly's lip tremble and realised now was the moment to exit.

"Right then Molly we had better get going if we are to get to the pet shop on time. We are going to collect Molly's Christmas present a few days early."

"How exciting!" exclaimed Mrs Carter, understanding the need to make the exit as easy as possible, "What are you having or is it a surprise?"

Molly lifted her head from its determined fix on Trixie and said softly, "A terrapin, Dad can't have fur in the house so this will be OK for him."

"How lovely! I understand they are friendly little creatures if you treat them right. I expect you will need lots of bits and pieces for the tank. Can I give you a little something to buy an ornament or two? I'd like to, as a thank you for letting us look after Trixie." She waved away Katie's burgeoning protest and reaching for her purse she extracted a ten-pound note. "There, that should help. You can tell me what you bought when you next come to visit."

Molly glanced at her mother to check it was Ok to accept. Katie nodded and Molly whispered a thank you. Then with a last look back at the little dog she grabbed her mother's hand and followed her through the door. Trixie went to join them, but Mrs Carter reached down and gently restrained her.

"You stay here my love; we will be taking care of you now."

Chapter 46

Christmas

December 2019

Christmas passed quietly for once. There was plenty of morning excitement which Katie carefully shielded her mother from, as too much noise and activity seemed to distress her these days. The children opened their stockings on their parent's bed as usual, then one present each was left under the tree for when Joan was awake. Joan smiled benignly as each present was unwrapped and exclaimed with delight over her own. Her favourite was a picture Molly had drawn of Trixie and put in a frame for her.

Molly's terrapin was a huge hit. She named him Bobi as he bobbed about and everyone was enchanted by the way he popped his head up out of the water, hoping for food, whenever anyone approached. His tank and all the accessories had cost a small fortune and Katie was aghast at the strict cleaning routine. However, Jack had reassured her he would take that on. He insisted it would be his father- daughter time. Katie wondered if he was feeling a little guilty over Molly's heartbreak over Trixie. Either way, she was happy to accept his offer.

They had shared a traditional Christmas lunch and spent the afternoon playing games together. The TV was on in the background and Joan had watched until she had nodded off. For once everything seemed peaceful. Katie knew that it was a temporary lull, yet she was grateful all the same.

On Boxing Day Jack and the girls set off to visit his parents. Matt had asked if he could be excused and join some friends at the cinema as one of them was celebrating his birthday. Poor kid had been born on Christmas Day and always struggled to have a separate celebration. Jack had grumbled, then accepted with good grace in the end. Katie was therefore left to spend the day with her mother.

She had decided to try to recreate something from her own childhood. As there had only been the two of them, they had developed their own unique little routines. One of those was that on Boxing Day Joan didn't cook, instead they went out for "high tea" as she had called it. This was at a lovely hotel near their home. When Katie had rung, she was absolutely delighted to discover they still offered a similar meal. It was 'afternoon tea' now, with more cakes and pastries and less sausage rolls and scotch eggs; lovely all the same. Joan had not been at all surprised when Katie told her where they were going.

"Well of course," she had said, "We always go there!"

It had been 20 years since they last had. However, Katie accepted her mother's reality was different to hers these days.

Joan insisted on wearing a smart skirt and blouse. Katie did likewise. Although she chuckled inwardly when her mother also found a hat. It had been hers once but had long since been surrendered to Molly for the dressing up box. Straw with a sunny yellow ribbon, it didn't quite belong in the depths of winter. However, Joan placed it on her head with a flourish as they set off.

Katie simply smiled as they caught a few curious glances when they entered the restaurant. Curious glances at a summer hat in December were not going to phase her one bit.

They were shown to their table and as the waiter handed them menus, Joan removed her hat, looking around anxiously for somewhere to put it.

"Shall I take that for you?" asked the waiter. "I can put it in the cloakroom if you want."

"Oh thank you said Joan. Can you take our coats too?" The waiter grinned and took it all.

They had a delightful meal. There were tiny sandwiches cut into triangles and buttery scones with miniature pots of jam and cream. Followed by a whole stand of tiny little cakes each. Katie chose two from her selection, while Joan happily munched her way through all of hers. The tea came in pots with old fashioned cosies and Joan was thrilled when the lovely waiter brought her a second pot. He winked at Katie as he poured her mother a steaming hot cup and replaced the cosy.

"There you go my love, that's really fresh."

"Thank you," smiled Joan.

"Thank you," mouthed Katie, meaning far more than just the tea.

"No problem," said the waiter, "you remind me of my nan."

"Do I know her?" asked Joan.

The waiter paused and shook his head softly.

"No, my love she didn't live around here. We lost her this time last year. She loved her tea and cakes though. Just like you. Now tuck in I don't want to see any crumbs left."

Joan smiled and turned back to her food. She loved having Katie to herself. And what a lovely place. It looked vaguely familiar, although it was not the place they usually went. Never mind the cakes were delicious.

Katie loved sitting there watching her mother enjoy herself. How she wished she had more time for moments like these. She vowed she would make it happen in the New Year.

They sat for almost three hours before they reluctantly got up to leave. Katie took her mother to the bathroom and then hovered outside waiting for her. The waiter who had served them was just cashing up a bill and she caught his eye. He grinned and stepped towards her.

"Everything OK?" he asked.

"More than OK, it has been amazing, thank you."

"No problem, just doing my job."

"Forgive me for asking, but your nan, was it…?"

"Alzheimer's, yes. Eight years it took to lose her bit by bit. Horrible."

"I'm sorry, it must be hard to see people like us come in."

"Oh no it's lovely. Lovely to see you enjoying yourselves. I used to take my nan out every Sunday to give Mum a break. I got all the fun; Mum did all the work. I wish Mum had been the one to go out sometimes and I had just taken a turn sitting with Nan. Mum's memories aren't too good now; she lost her warmth in dealing with all the tough stuff. If I had any advice, it would be to make sure you keep enjoying times like today. These moments, they are precious. The rest, well it's just hard."

Katie swallowed and smiled again.

"I will," she whispered. "I will."

Chapter 47

Carers

Joan froze. She could hear someone moving about downstairs. It was still dark. She closed her eyes and hoped the noises would stop. Why wasn't Trixie barking? It was no good, there was definitely someone in her house. They were in the kitchen. She listened carefully to try to make out what they were doing. It sounded like the kettle. Why would someone break into her house and use the kettle? The fridge opened. Perhaps a homeless person had broken in and was hungry. Should she be worried? Perhaps they would just take food and then leave? No, the footsteps were in the hall now. They were coming up the stairs. She pulled her covers up over her head and hid.

"Good morning Joan!"

Joan stayed firmly under the covers. She did not know that voice.

"I've got a cup of tea for you. I'll pop it here while I get things ready for your wash. Let's pull back the curtains, shall we? Can you pop your head out for me? Joan sweetheart it's morning."

Slowly Joan slid the covers down until her eyes peeped out. She stared at the strange woman bustling about in her room. She was a middle-aged black lady with short tight curls and glasses. She wore a white apron over a blue dress. She didn't look homeless. Or dangerous and she had come armed only with a cup of tea. Joan pulled the covers off her head and looked about her. The woman was taking clothes out of her drawers now and looking in her wardrobe.

"That's it let's sit you up so you can drink your tea." Now the woman was pulling her upright. Handing her a cup of tea. Joan took it, took one sip. It tasted alright. Although why was this woman here?

"Right then, you drink that and I will sort out the bathroom for your wash. Then we will get you dressed and downstairs for breakfast."

"But who are you? And why are you in my bedroom?"

"Oh sweetheart I'm Elaine. I'm your morning call. I came last week a couple of times. I've not had you on my roster since. The agency likes to keep us all on our toes I think, switching us around. Now drink up and let's get you sorted."

Joan frowned. Somewhere in the mists she remembered. There were people who came now. People who gave her food and moved her about. Perhaps it was because she banged her knee. She smiled. This one seemed kind enough.

"Yes of course you are. Sorry I wasn't quite awake."

Once Elaine had gone, Joan realised she was still tired. She was downstairs now with the TV on and a bowl of cornflakes on a tray in front of her. She wasn't hungry. It was still dark outside. The streetlights were still on. She put the tray on the coffee table and got up. She went over to the stairs. There was that lift thing. She wouldn't bother with that. Slowly, carefully, one step at a time she made her way back to her bedroom. Her knee ached. She pulled back the covers and lay down. She would just take a little nap.

Katie was looking at the call book. She had popped in at lunchtime hoping to catch the carer so she could see how her mum interacted with them. It was almost 2.00 pm and she had been there over an hour. According to the log, breakfast had been at 6.00am. Katie had found the congealing cornflakes in the living room and her mother stranded upstairs. She was washed and dressed but complaining that her knee hurt. Katie had painstakingly shown her how to use the stairlift yet again, although it was obvious her mother could not manage it alone. She had made her a sandwich and a cup of tea and sat with her while she ate it.

A loud screeching noise came from the kitchen making them both jump. Joan looked terrified and put a cushion up in front of her face.

"It's alright Mum it is just the pill pot. It's telling you it is time to take your medicine."

"Make it stop!" pleaded Joan. "I don't like that noise!"

Katie fetched the pot and showed Joan for the umpteenth time how to turn it over, so the correct pills fell out and the noise stopped.

"There I will get you some water to take them."

While Katie was in the kitchen, the front door opened and a new voice called out.

"Hello!"

Katie returned to the living room and stood a little back from the door to watch her mother's reaction.

Joan looked up at the woman. She was tall and thin with long brown hair. She looked as though she was in her mid-twenties. She wore a blue dress and a white apron. She shook her head slowly. No, she had no idea who this person was. Katie was here though so it would all be OK. She smiled at the stranger.

The woman spoke with a heavy Eastern European accent.

"Joan you make your own sandwich? How clever. And a cup of tea. I told you not touch that kettle or you burn yourself. Is it fresh? You like another?"

Joan beamed. "Yes please."

"OK I make one and I cook your meal for you?"

"Thank you," said Joan.

"OK what is it today. I will look in the freezer. You want meat or fish?"

"I don't mind, whatever you think," smiled Joan.

The carer headed for the kitchen, almost bumping into Katie.

"Oh hello. Who are you?"

"I'm Katie, Joan's daughter."

"Pleased to meet you. I am Agnetha. Her lunchtime call for today. I go cook her dinner."

"She has just had a sandwich. She won't want dinner."

"But I cook for her now. I have only 15 minutes. Next visit much later. She need it now or be hungry. Unless you stay and cook later?"

"I have to go soon. I have been here over an hour. I found Mum dressed upstairs but her breakfast was downstairs. She can't do the stairlift herself. The log says the carer came at 6.00 am and now it is nearly 2.00. Mum had had nothing to eat and why was she left upstairs like that?

"I don't know. I not do morning. You ring agency perhaps?"

"Why are you so late?"

"I not late. This my time. Look here my call sheet." The woman pulled a piece of paper out of her apron pocket. Sure enough, among the many names, there was her mother's with the time listed as 2.00pm."

"But her breakfast was at 6.00 am. That is far too long."

"I not do planning, I just visit. I need cook now or I be late for next visit."

Katie sighed. Perhaps her mother was hungry enough to eat the meal. She had to go soon to be on time to collect Lucy from school. At best she could stay another 30 minutes, although she had intended to pick up some fresh vegetables to go with their chicken that evening. She looked around her. She had loaded her mum's washing machine when she arrived. It was almost on the spin cycle. If she stayed until it was done, she would never get to the shops. Perhaps Agnetha would pop the clothes into the tumble dryer before she left? The girl was just taking the meal out of the freezer and popping it into the microwave.

"Look I really need to get on. This washing will be done in about ten minutes, could you pop it in the tumble dryer for me?"

Agnetha turned. She smiled at Katie but said firmly.

"That not my job."

"I know that. It is just I need to get to the shops and pick up my children."

"My job to cook, take your mum to toilet. Make sure she clean and talk with her. Give her company. Not do housework."

Katie sighed. "I have done your job. I've fed Mum and talked to her for over an hour. She isn't hungry for the food you are cooking and she has just been to the toilet, which is actually something she can do alone. Her clothes were dirty and she won't put them in the dryer herself. It will only take a minute and would be really helpful."

Agnetha took the dinner out of the microwave and placed the plastic tray onto a plate. She rummaged in the drawer for a knife and fork and then turned to Katie.

"I must do my job. That the rules. I must write in log. My boss check. I be late, I lose wages unless good reason. Washing not good reason. I give this Joan now. Then I must go."

She turned and went through to Joan. "There you go Joan. Nice fish pie."

"Thank you." Joan picked up the knife and fork and started to eat. "Lovely!" she said.

Later that evening as Katie was busy cooking, while simultaneously helping Molly with some tricky maths homework, the phone rang. It was the care agency. She realised she had forgotten to ring them so grabbed her phone while urgently asking Molly to take over stirring the pan.

"Mrs Robinson, It's Tracey from Kind Smiles Carers here. Do you have a minute to talk?"

"Yes, I was going to call you actually I'm…"

"Good well we were a little worried today when one of our carers called to say you were asking her to do domestic tasks. Those are not her responsibility. She has limited time and her role is to care for your mother."

Katie fumed inwardly, while speaking softly, "I appreciate what you are saying but…"

Again, Tracey cut her off, "Good I'm glad you understand. If you do need domestic help, we have a group of excellent cleaners, who also do washing and ironing. Our rates are very competitive."

"We have a cleaner thank you. I am worried Mum is…"

"Ok that's good. Sorry I must go as I have another call coming in. Have a nice evening. Goodbye."

Katie starred at the phone. The social worker had promised her this agency provided high quality care delivered with compassion. Their website trumpeted their individualised packages. Katie's eyes had watered at the prices they charged and was grateful Joan qualified for free help. Perhaps that was it she thought. Perhaps you got second rate if you were state subsidised. She resolved to take her concerns to the social worker. Right now

though, she needed to rescue the sauce Molly had diligently
stirred but not recognised as done.

Chapter 48

More carers

January 2020

"Hello, who are you?" Joan smiled and the lady coming in through her door. She was short and round with curls that bounced as she walked.

"I'm Milly," she smiled. "I'm here to make you some lunch."

"Oh that's kind of you. But I'm not hungry. Shall we just have a cup of tea instead?"

"If that's what you would prefer my love then I'll pop the kettle on."

Joan and Milly sat sharing their tea while Joan regaled Milly with her favourite tales of her childhood. Milly laughed in all the right places and nodded appreciatively at Joan's anecdotes.

"Well, it has been lovely chatting to you Joan. Now are you sure I can't make you some food before I go?"

"Oh no I'm not at all hungry. Do you have to leave so soon?"

Milly glanced at her watch. She had a 30 minute break coming up before going to that bad tempered Mr Walters. Sitting here in Joan's nice warm house was lovely. She had no pressing errand to run in her break and it wasn't long enough to go home.

"I guess I can stay a few more minutes. Shall I refresh the pot?"

"Lovely, "said Joan.

Joan looked in the fridge. There was a block of cheese, some tomatoes and cucumber in there. And milk. She opened the cupboard. Some tins of soup and baked beans. The freezer was full of those horrible frozen meals Katie kept buying. Nothing tasty anywhere. She picked up her coat and headed for the door. She would just pop to the shops and get something nice to eat.

Maybe some eggs. She could scramble them later. First, she would have some biscuits. Nice chocolate ones. They had her favourites in the local shop.

Thirty minutes later and Joan had tucked into a packet of penguins followed by a bowl of raspberry ripple ice cream. It had been on special offer in the shop and she just thought it would slip down nicely. She had followed it all up with a glass of wine from the bottle she had treated herself to. There were eggs in the fridge. She would scramble them later. Now, now she was going to have a little nap.

"Mummy Grandma is still in bed!"

"What do you mean Lucy. Is she awake or sleeping?" Katie had dropped Matt at football and Molly with a friend before going over to her mother's house to check on her. Lucy had been happy to come as she wanted to sing a new song she had learnt at school to her grandmother. They were already preparing for the Easter service and Lucy seemed to have forgotten how Grandma had ruined the last one. Katie had opened the door and been diverted by an odd smell from the kitchen. Lucy had run upstairs to see her grandmother.

"She's awake and she's dressed but she is in bed."

Katie had found the source of the smell. Yesterday's dinner was sitting on the table untouched. It was some kind of chicken dish covered in a garlic sauce. She scooped it up and took it out to the dustbin. Then she opened the windows wide to let out the smell. The kitchen needed a good scrub. The cleaner was either getting less efficient or the varied carers were not clearing up behind themselves. Dishes were piled in the sink along with far too many tea mugs. Others were scattered around the house, half drunk and then abandoned.

"Are you coming up Mummy?"

Katie cast one last look at the mess and went upstairs.

"Hello Mum, what are you doing in bed in your clothes?" She realised as she said it that the question was pointless, as Joan wouldn't remember the answer.

"Oh I'm just having a rest."

"Are you tired still Mum?"

"No, I'm hungry. And thirsty."

"Haven't you had breakfast?"

"Is it time for breakfast?"

Katie smiled and took her mother's hand. "Come on Mum let's see what we can find for you. Lucy, can you go ride the stair lift up here so Grandma can go down on it please." Lucy skipped off gleefully while Katie mused on the fact that while her little child could work the machine, her mother had no clue.

Once they were downstairs and Joan was happily tucking into scrambled eggs made with some mysterious eggs Katie was sure she hadn't bought, washed down with a glass of orange juice, Katie picked up the log. She saw that the last visit, the day before, had been at 6.30. That was just one hour after the dinner visit. The log noted that Joan refused to get ready for bed, so the carer gave her a cup of tea and left her watching television. The dinner visit said Joan had not been there when she arrived, so the meal had been prepared and left on the table. The agency had been called to alert them that Joan was missing. Lunchtime had been at 12.30 but Joan had refused lunch and insisted she would make her own. The carer had made a cup of tea and left her to it.

Katie started turning back over previous pages. Repeatedly she saw that her mother had refused food saying she would make her own. The timings of visits were haphazard and the writing so varied it was clear it was rarely the same person. So far no one had visited that day. She looked carefully at her mother. Her hair was standing on end and she was pretty sure she had been wearing those clothes the day before. She feared Joan had slept in her clothes. How had she got up the stairs? The lift was firmly at the bottom when they arrived.

As she pondered what to do next the front door opened and in came a harassed looking girl with bright pink hair dragging a toddler behind her.

"Oh crap!" she exclaimed when she saw Katie and Lucy sitting there with Joan.

"Sorry I shouldn't have said that. Please don't tell."

"I've heard worse," said Joan, "Now who do we have here?" She smiled benevolently at the girl and the little child.

Katie had been so shocked by their arrival that she hadn't responded. Joan's reaction had now wrong footed her.

"Yes, who do we have here?" she asked in a softer tone than she would have.

"My name is Sam and this is my son Ethan. He's supposed to be with his dad, who should have picked him up an hour ago. I managed to get my mate Jen to cover the rest of my calls. She works for the same agency so it's OK," she added when she saw the alarm on Katie's face. "We cover each other a lot at the weekends, as we both have little ones with dodgy dads who don't always turn up on time. But this call was too early for her as her kid's dad wasn't due till 11.00 and I was worried about Joan as I'm her first visit and I know she can't do the stairs and so I thought it would be OK to bring him along just this once. Joan always talks about her grandchildren. You must be Lucy?"

All of this tumbled out in a rush and then the girl stood breathless, staring at Katie. Katie stared back, unsure of how to proceed.

"Please don't tell, "whispered the girl, "It's a sackable offence. This is my first proper job. I don't want to go back on the social. I like earning. Means Ethan and I can get on a bit..." she tailed off, as Katie still stood, silent.

"Lucy why don't you find the little boy a chocolate biscuit." piped up Joan. "Then we can all have a nice cup of tea. Katie, can you put the kettle on?"

"Just a minute Mum. Yes, Lucy find a biscuit for the little boy. Sam you and I are going into a different room for a minute."

She led the way into the living room and gestured for Sam to sit down.

"First off, I am not going to report you. I've fed Mum and I will get her into the bath and change her clothes. I appreciate this mess is not your fault. However, poor Mum was upstairs in the same clothes she wore yesterday- she slept in them I believe- with nothing to eat or drink. In return I want some information about your agency from you. I want to understand a bit better how things work."

"Ok, but you won't tell it came from me?"

"No."

"My mother's rota is so haphazard it makes me confused and I don't have dementia. Goodness knows what it feels like for her. For instance, why on earth was her bedtime visit at 6.30 last night?"

"I didn't do that one."

"I appreciate that, but is it normal to put someone to bed so early? And then what time were you due this morning?"

"10.00am."

Katie glanced at her watch. "So you were actually only half an hour late. That means my mum was supposed to be in bed from 6.30 last night until 10 this morning. Who plans these things?"

"I dunno exactly. Your mum is what the office calls an 'add on'."

"A what?"

"We all have our regulars. Least we share them. They're the paying customers. They have 3 or 4 of us who visit them and their times are quite set. Some of the socials get treated the same. If they stick that is. Often though we are just a short-term thing before they go into a home. So, then they are an add on. They fit their visits round the regulars whenever someone is free. It's particularly bad like that in the first 6 weeks. While the social are assessing exactly what they need. If your mum sticks it will get more regular."

"But not like a paying customer though?"

"I dunno, I've probably said too much. But you know how it is. The agencies wanna keep the rich people. There will always be plenty from the socials and they don't get to choose how things is done. But the rich ones, well they have other agencies to choose from."

"Do you mind me asking what you are paid?"

Sam shrugged. "£8.50 an hour."

"Do you know what the agency charge?"

"Yeah, I looked it up on my phone. £30 a visit."

"What do they do for their share."

"They run the office and stuff. I dunno. I'm new, they tell me I might earn more if I work for a year for them. And do some training."

"OK Sam, I really appreciate what you have told me. I promise I won't get you into trouble."

"Thanks. I really appreciate it."

"Now let's go see if our children have polished off all the biscuits!"

As they walked to the kitchen Sam ventured a question of her own.

"Do you think your mum will stick? Only I like coming here and hoped she might be one of my regulars. She's lovely and kind…."

Katie didn't reply. Her look said it all.

After Sam had left, Katie helped her mother wash and dress in clean clothes. She gathered up the dirty ones to take home and put in her own family wash. She washed up the dirty dishes and wiped down the worst of the kitchen surfaces. She knew the cleaner would be in on Monday and she was going to keep her mother home with her for the weekend. Last of all she rang the agency.

"Hello, it's Katie Robinson here, Joan Jessup's daughter. Just to let you know Mum is staying with me for the rest of the weekend so won't need any visits. Until Monday morning."

"That's a bit too short notice we need 24…"

"Sorry, family emergency, goodbye." Katie grimaced. She would deal with them later. First, she had to deal with Jack and the social worker.

Lucy was very excited that Grandma was coming home to play. She chattered to her all the way there. Joan was a bit bemused, while happy to be going anywhere with her beloved granddaughter. That gave Katie time to think and to formulate a plan.

As they walked through the door Jack spotted the overnight bag and gave Katie a quizzical look. He waited until Joan and Lucy were happily playing dressing up in the playroom before he spoke.

"I thought you were just visiting your mother. We had plans for today. Remember? We have a babysitter booked so we can go out to dinner with my new client."

Katie had forgotten that. "We can still go. I'll make sure Mum is ready for bed the same as the children. She will just sit and watch TV. It will be fine. I couldn't leave her there. You don't understand how awful it was."

Then for once, just like that, Katie burst into tears.

Jack rearranged his client dinner using the excuse of a family emergency. It was one after all he told Katie. Then they talked through options. Jack was keen to try again with the care but felt it was important to speak to those in authority about the difficulties Joan had been experiencing. In the meantime, they would start looking at care homes. Joan's house would be put on the market to pay for it. He would speak to an estate agent on Monday. Katie would tackle the social worker and then, if necessary, the care company. She hoped the social worker would deal with them for her.

Joan had a lovely weekend playing with Lucy and was quite loathe to return home on Sunday evening. Katie tucked her into bed as she would one of her children, kissing her gently on her forehead as she smoothed down her blankets.

"Sleep tight Mum. I will pop back tomorrow after work. You will have lots of visitors to cook for you and a trip out to your singing club."

"Is Katy coming?"

Katie shook her head a bit bemused at the question.

"Yes, yes I told you I would come. After work."

Joan shrugged and closed her eyes. Katie slipped downstairs. She had left notes for the carers to make sure her mother was left a cold meal if she refused to eat when they were there. And that under no circumstances was she to be left stranded upstairs. That was all she could do from this end. She needed to tackle the root of the problem.

Chapter 49

Reality

January 2020

On Monday morning Katie put a call through to the social worker in charge of her case. She got a secretary who tried to fob her off with a ring back later as she had back-to-back meetings all morning. Jack had coached her well on how to get past secretaries, so she summoned her most authoritative voice and said, "I don't think you quite appreciate the seriousness of the situation. I think if Miss Jones discovers you didn't get my message to her and there is no resolution of the current difficulties, she will be very concerned that you have obstructed an important outcome." It sounded like nonsense to Katie, although Jack had assured her it worked every time.

It did. The secretary hesitated a second and then put Katie on hold. A tense moment later and she heard Miss Jones' imperious tones.

"What is it that is so vital? I have come out of a very important meeting to take this call."

Katie took a breath.

"I believe the care company are mistreating my mother." Again, Jack had coached her in the vocabulary she should use.

"In what way?"

"I would like to discuss that in person. Please know I had to remove my mother from their care for the weekend for her safety."

There was a pause and then, "Can you be here today at 5.00pm?"

"Yes."

"Please bring the logbook."

Katie's headmistress had covered her class so she could make the call. Following it, she had a busy day of teaching. She raced off afterwards to collect her girls, dropping them home with Jack who had for once pulled out all the stops to help her and was working from home. He had even ordered take away in advance for dinner. Then she dashed across town to check on her mum and collect the logbook. Joan was happily watching a gardening programme with a fresh cup of tea by her chair, and a slice of cake. When Katie enquired about the cake she was told "Katy made it," so she shrugged and decided to just be grateful her mother was happy. She knew the logbook wasn't supposed to leave the house, so she removed one blank page for the later carers to fill in, just in case she didn't get it back in time. Then she left to make her 5.00pm meeting.

She ran breathless up the stairs just after 5.05 clutching the logbook. She was greeted by the secretary who showed her haughtily into a side room before telling her Miss Jones would be along soon as she had been held up by an emergency. Katie took the delay as time to go over her planned approach once more. By the time Miss Jones arrived she was sure she knew exactly what to say. The social worker's first words stopped her in her tracks.

"Right as your allegation is so serious, I have asked the head of the care company to join us. She will be here in half an hour. First, I would like you to outline to me the case for mistreatment."

Katie faltered realising that in her determination to be heard she had overdone things. She took a breath and decided her mother still needed her to speak out. Calmly and clearly she outlined the ways she had found her mother, not fed, not dressed, sleeping in her clothes, food left to congeal. None of it was life threatening but all of it added up to a poor picture of care. She showed how many times the log said her mother didn't eat. She explained about all the abandoned mugs and plates. In short, she described a pattern of neglect.

Miss Jones listened intently. At the end she asked only one question.

"Has your mother shown any signs of injury?"

"No…"

Miss Jones sighed. "Look I do appreciate how hard this is. Quite frankly I think your mother needs more care than she is getting. Full time care. We can't offer that at the moment, although as I have explained before a care home package might be available out of area. We can improve some things. We can make sure carers know you want meals left for your mother even if she turns them down. I can ask for more stable visits and for more consistent carers. I would suggest putting a bed downstairs and blocking off the stairs, although as you have no washing facilities downstairs that would make it harder. It's not unmanageable; a carer could take her up to wash and back down to sleep. You should also seriously consider fitting a dishwasher. Carers don't wash up; they don't have time. However, they will put things in a dishwasher. Once it is full, they will turn it on. The one part of your tale that bothers me most is that your mother wasn't there during a visit for no planned reason and while it was logged no one alerted you or me. If she went out alone once I would imagine she is doing it more often. And while we can't lock her in, we do need to be concerned about that. What happened to the alarm?"

"We turned it off," admitted Katie somewhat sheepishly. "It kept going off when Mum opened the door for visitors, the people who take her to activities especially, and they didn't know how to stop it. It was such a nuisance…" she trailed off.

"You realise many of those we care for have no visitors. They spend their lives sitting at home waiting for their carers to arrive. No family, no friends, no outings. Your mother is much more fortunate than many."

Katie sighed. "I do…but she is my mum and she is the one I need to look out for. And it isn't right that she is suffering this way."

Miss Jones paused and then unexpectedly reached out and patted Katie's arm.

"I agree. Nothing about this is fair or right. This government was elected partly on a pledge to fix social care. So far nothing has happened and if the rumours of an impending pandemic prove true nothing will. I have spent half of today dealing with a man whose house is rammed so full of his 'collections' he can no longer get out the front door. There are rats running around among the abandoned food cartons and his skin is peeling off due to so many sores from not being washed. No one has visited him in years and it was only when the postman couldn't get any more mail through the door that we were alerted. I'm absolutely not saying your mother doesn't deserve better. She does. We all do. But sadly, I have to prioritise the worst cases and your mother is far from that."

Chastened Katie bowed her head for a moment before remembering why she came.

"I only have my mother to worry about. I can't leave her like this."

"I understand. You will have to find an alternative then. Look why don't you go now before the care company manager arrives. I will explain there was a misunderstanding and try to get some tweaks to the arrangements. You go home and talk to your family. Then call me when you have a plan."

"Thank you," said Katie meekly, although deep down she knew that all Miss Jones had done was hand the problem back to her.

It only took a week. The estate agent had given a good value for the house as long as it was cleaned up a bit as he put it. Jack arranged professional cleaners to do what they could and decorators to give the place a lick of paint. Katie packed up all Joan's personal items and put them in her loft. Joan and her clothes moved back into the playroom. Matt's old room became a shared space for the girls, and he got his dream of moving into the room over the garage. Ostensibly Joan was to stay until the house was sold and then a suitable care home found. No one really believed that would happen. Katie took a leave of absence from work for the rest of term and resigned going forward. She loved her job, but she loved her mother more.

Chapter 50

Katy's Goodbye

January 2020

"Hello? Joan are you in?" Katy knocked again on the door but there was still no answer. The dog wasn't barking either. She shook her head slowly. Trixie hadn't been there the last few times Katy had seen Joan and when she asked about her Joan had been vague. In the past Joan had occasionally been out when she called, although never two weeks in a row. Except the time when Joan had hurt her knee. Katy knew nothing of the accident then, only that her friend wasn't there when she called. She had continued to drop by every Friday in the hope that Joan would return. Briefly she had considered tracking down Joan's daughter, then decided not to intrude. Relieved when Joan reappeared, she had surmised from her friend's indistinct comments that the injury had meant a stay with her family. This felt different though. The house looked different. Cold and empty.

She thought about the last time she had seen Joan. Something hadn't been right. Joan had appeared slightly sweaty, and her breathing wasn't right. She seemed more confused than ever and kept asking Katy when she would be moving. Katy had no idea about any moving plans and kept trying to reassure the old lady she didn't have to go anywhere. However, Joan kept wanting to pack. In the end they found an old case and put some of her clothes into it. Katy carefully folding each of the musty jumpers pulled from a drawer that clearly hadn't been opened in a while. As they packed Joan rattled on about the happy years spent in her house with her husband and child. She didn't want to leave them behind, even though she knew she had to go now. She didn't seem to know where. Katy thought of calling the doctor.

However, when she asked Joan if she would like her to, Joan just laughed. She said she had seen the doctor, the smiling one, she couldn't remember why. Katie said it was all OK and she mustn't worry, she just had to pack. It was a difficult visit all round and in some ways, Katy had been glad to leave. If only she had known, it would be the last.

She decided to investigate further. She tried the garden gate, unusually it was open. She walked round to the back noticing the weeds had been pulled from all the cracks between the slabs along the side of the house. The bushes were all neatly pruned too. Her eyes swept the back garden. It looked neat, even professionally tidy. All the randomly placed pots were gone and the usual chair where Joan liked to sit to catch the sun was missing. Katy blinked back tears. Had her friend really left? She glanced into the kitchen through the patio doors. Everywhere was polished and gleaming. All traces of Joan erased.

Katy paused, her heart pounding. She wasn't sure what this meant. Perhaps Joan had gone to live with her daughter permanently. Whatever would she do without Joan's company? Waves of loss crashed over her and she gasped for air. She shook herself firmly. This isn't the same, she could find Joan again. What clues did she have? Her daughter was a teacher, that much she knew for certain. And she had grandchildren, the youngest was called Lucy. If only she could remember the name of the school where they had found Lucy. That first day when Joan had turned up looking for her in the wrong place. Katy smiled, remembering the confused old lady she had insisted on helping. How the secretary had frowned at her! It had become a precious part of her week, visiting Joan. What fun they had had dancing round the living room together that time! Katy smiled to herself. That experience had triggered a change in her own life. Joan's enthusiasm had inspired her to take herself along to a local dance group. Now she took part in ballroom dance each week and had even been invited to enter a competition in a few months' time. She was enjoying the company of the other dancers. One of the girls, Susie, had asked her to meet for coffee after work on a Friday. Katy had apologised, explaining about Joan and how she had to see her instead. Susie had shrugged and moved on, a little put out it seemed. Perhaps next week she would meet Susie if the offer still stood.

Katy looked around her once more. She knew she wouldn't come back. Clearly Joan was gone. She nodded slowly, recognising that for a time they had helped each other, but that time was over. She took a breath. She wasn't losing Joan; she was letting her go. There was a difference.

Chapter 51

Going to the Park

February 2020

Katie was sorting washing. She seemed to spend at least a quarter of her life doing washing. She was upstairs putting clothes back into the right rooms. As she put Molly's things neatly into her drawer, she reflected on how well it was going having her mum live with them. One more at the dinner table wasn't a problem really and the children, especially Lucy, seemed to regard Joan as an extra child to play with and Joan was more than happy to oblige them. Once they had put a television in Joan's room, so she didn't intrude on Jack's evening viewing, even he was mollified. She glanced out the window where Lucy was playing with a ball while Joan looked on smiling benignly. Yes, it had definitely been a good decision. Far better than the endless panicked dashes across town. Or the disastrous carers.

Lucy was playing in the garden. It was a rare sunny day for the time of year. Grandma was watching her bounce her ball. She could catch it most of the time now. Grandma was counting the bounces. She kept missing out numbers and that just made Lucy giggle. It was all part of the game.

Joan was happy too. It was warm in Katie's pretty garden and she loved being trusted to care for Lucy. She wasn't losing her marbles after all. Not if she could take care of a child.

"Grandma can we go to the park?"

Joan hesitated. Wasn't there a reason she shouldn't leave the house? She was looking after Lucy so it must be OK. She would just tell Katie they were going. She turned to go indoors. Lucy had already opened the gate.

"Lucy wait!" She hurried after her.

Katie glanced back out of the window. She couldn't see Joan or Lucy. Maybe they had come indoors. She listened. She could hear movement downstairs. She went back to putting clothes away.

Joan wasn't sure which was the right way to the park. She tried to hold Lucy's hand, but Lucy was bouncing the ball. Lucy was walking too quickly. Joan couldn't keep up. Something wasn't right. There was something she wasn't supposed to do.

"Slow down Lucy I'm not sure of the way," she said.

"I know the way Grandma. We just walk along this path and then cross the road and we are at the park."

That was it! She wasn't to cross the road on her own. Katie had said it wasn't safe.

"Lucy love, I'm not supposed to cross the road. It isn't safe you know."

"It's OK Grandma I'm not allowed to either! Except at the zebra crossing. So we can go there can't we? It's right opposite the park."

Joan still wasn't sure. There was another reason she had to stay home wasn't there? Lucy was skipping ahead again bouncing her ball along the pavement. She hurried to catch up.

Katie had finished putting the clothes away and headed downstairs. Matt and Molly were in the living room. Molly was absorbed in drawing while Matt was watching TV.

"Where are Lucy and Grandma? I thought they came in?"

"Huh?" muttered Matt

"Grandma? Lucy?" Have you seen them?

"Nah!"

"Molly? Have you?"

"Sorry Mum have I what?"

"Seen Lucy and Grandma?"

"They are playing outside I think."

Katie opened the back door. Neither Lucy nor Joan was in the garden. The gate was open. She started to run.

Lucy was excited. Mummy never had time to take her to the park these days. Since Grandma moved, in Mummy seemed to spend lots more time washing and cooking. The park wasn't far, although she knew she shouldn't go alone. She hadn't had she? Grandma was a grown up so that was OK. She had a little nagging feeling that she ought to have asked Mummy first. Then again Grandma said she was going to tell Mummy didn't she, so it must be OK.

Lucy and Joan reached the zebra crossing.

"We need to look both ways," said Joan carefully. It's right first and then left. Or maybe left first. You have to do one of them twice. She frowned. Which was it?

"It's OK Grandma it's a zebra crossing. The cars have to stop for people silly!"

Joan saw the car before Lucy did.

Chapter 52

Definitions

February 21st 2020

"I am the Lord of the Dance said he…" the congregation were mumbling the words all wrong. It had seemed like a good choice for the hymn. After all it was Lucy's favourite and it had been so joyous when Joan had joined in at the Easter service at school. Now it jarred and no one felt like dancing. Katie twisted her hankie round and round in her fingers. She looked at Jack standing next to her staring blankly ahead not singing a word. She reached for his hand, but he was holding the hymn book. She tucked her arm in his, needing him to steady her. He looked at her quizzically; what did she expect if she chose such a stupid hymn for a funeral.

The vicar told them to sit. Molly was next to her. She had tears in her eyes and Katie reached to wipe them. She looked at Matt, sitting bolt upright like his dad, determined to show no emotion. A shudder ran through her. The vicar droned on; Katie wasn't listening; she just kept twisting her hankie.

"And now we have a few words from Katie."

Katie felt her legs wobble as she walked to the front. She stood for a second behind the lectern. Her eyes took in the congregation. She saw one of Lucy's friend's mums in the back row, next to an elderly man she vaguely remembered and the kind teacher from the school Mum once wandered into. What was her name? Oh yes Katy Bishop. Fancy her coming. That man what was his name?

Everyone was looking at her. She knew she had to start but she couldn't think what she was supposed to say. She looked at Jack for help. Wordlessly he handed her the paper she had been scrawling on all night. Eulogies needed to be personal she had told him fiercely. Written by those who truly loved the person. Delivering it, that was a different story. She decided to focus on the back row. She couldn't look at Matt or Molly. She caught the eye of Katy Bishop who gave her an encouraging smile. She smoothed her paper, smoothed her skirt, cleared her throat, opened her mouth, still the words were stuck inside.

She realised who the elderly man was, it was Billy, Joan's childhood playmate of sorts. She tried again. Then she noticed two strangers along the row with pens poised. Her family tragedy had made front page news in the local rag and even warranted a few lines in one of the daily tabloids. Anger seethed, she put the paper to one side and at last she started to speak.

"Much has been said in recent days about my family. Some true, some not. Lots of opinions and speculation about what happened in one moment, on one day." She saw Jack shuffling in his seat no longer cool and detached.

"No one's life should be defined by one final moment. That is created by the many moments leading up to it. When my mother was a little girl, she had a neighbour called Billy. He's here today and I apologise if I embarrass him, but I need to tell this story. One day she found Billy teasing a tiny, defenceless kitten. She must have been about 5 at the time and he was 8, older, bigger, stronger. With all the righteous indignation of a child, she told him to stop, picked up the kitten and took it home. It stayed in her family for the rest of its days. I believe her mum had a few words with his, and one way or another he learnt his lesson. When Mum started school, it was Billy who walked protectively by her side to make sure she arrived safely.

Mum had a hideous disease. She no longer knew what day it was, forgot people's faces and where she was going. Her memories were fading one by one. Yet at her core she was still the same person who protected that kitten. My mum's last act on this earth was to step in front of a car to protect the little girl she adored. Because while Alzheimer's had robbed her of so very much it had not changed who she was. She loved Lucy, she saved her, and for that I will always be grateful."

Lucy was staring out the window when Katie finally went up to tuck her in. Her arm was still in a cast and it was itchy. Mummy's friend Jackie had been kind all day, but she wanted her mummy. She had wanted to go to say goodbye to Grandma too, though she didn't really know why she had to. No one was explaining much and she had been kept indoors out of sight of the odd people who kept ringing the doorbell. She had had to talk to a policeman and Daddy had looked cross. Mummy just kept hugging her and telling her it wasn't her fault. She knew that. The car was supposed to stop.

"Where's Grandma gone Mummy?"

Katie stopped, knowing of all the things she said today this would be the most important. And yet she wasn't sure herself. She followed Lucy's gaze out of the window.

She sat down on the bed.

"I'm not sure exactly sweetheart and that's the truth. Some people will tell you she has gone to Heaven. I hope that is true and that it is a beautiful place."

"But where is it Mummy?"

"Up past the stars in a faraway place."

"Can we visit?"

"No, we can't."

"I need to tell Grandma something."

Katie looked carefully at Lucy's scrunched up face.

"Can you tell me?"

"No, it needs to be Grandma."

"Wait there."

Katie went back downstairs and came back with a photograph. It had been taken at the school fete. Lucy and Grandma laughing together. She was planning to frame it and put it in Lucy's room as a keepsake.

"I don't think Grandma is up in the stars sweetheart. I think she is here inside of us. Everything she ever was, has been passed down in little bits to me and to you. When we need to talk to Grandma, we just need to look at her picture and think with our hearts what she would say and we will know that she still loves us. Wherever she has gone she's still here."

Lucy looked at the picture. Then she looked at her mother.

"Can you leave. This is just between me and Grandma."

Katie flinched but quietly left the room.

Lucy starred at the happy, smiling faces in the picture. She concentrated hard and then spoke out loud.

"I hope it's nice up in the stars in Heaven Grandma. I'm sorry I wanted to go to the park and that stupid car hit you. I miss playing with you, you were the best fun. They wouldn't let me come to say goodbye today, so I have to say it now."

Silent outside the door Katie watched Lucy plant a soft kiss on her grandma's face, then place the photo carefully by her bed, turn out her light and lie down to sleep.

Katie walked slowly down the stairs. She knew Lucy would recover. Not just physically, but emotionally too as she had all the resilience of a young child. And thankfully the memories would fade as she grew. The same was true for Matt and Molly. As for herself…the police had placed the blame squarely on the shoulders of the young speeding driver, but she… She caught sight of her favourite family photo. There they were all of them. Her three children, Jack not frowning for once, her not looking harassed and her mum, sitting in the middle grinning broadly at the centre of her world, her family. She paused, stared into her mother's eyes, and softly smiled back.

Epilogue

One Year Later

February 2021

Katie took a breath as she stepped through the archway into the Churchyard. She had wanted to come alone to sit quietly by her mother's grave and talk to her as she had so often in the last year. However, Lucy had overheard her telling Jack she intended to go and had insisted on coming too. She had accepted her daughter's need to do something to mark the anniversary and while she winced as Lucy snatched up some of the tiny snowdrops growing in their garden to add to Katie's shop brought roses, she knew in her heart which her mother would prefer. Lucy had chattered all the way to the Churchyard, an endless list of excited thoughts to share with Grandma. Now they were here she clutched her mother's hand in subdued silence.

Katie's thoughts meandered over the last year. Her mother had died just weeks before the Covid 19 pandemic hit the UK. While she missed her mother terribly, she knew from Maddy and Jackie how horrific care had been during that crisis. All the activities that had enriched their lives had stopped and they had had to keep their loved ones home. Jackie had lost her mother to the disease early on as it swept through care homes unchecked. Maddy's husband had deteriorated massively due to the lack of stimulation as he was trapped at home. She had been too afraid to move him to a care home. Instead, she battled on daily, washing, dressing and feeding the man she loved, who no longer recognised her or even acknowledged her efforts. While Katie could never say she was glad her mother was gone, she was grateful to have been spared that.

Katie had not returned to work after her mother's death. In the immediate aftermath she had desperately tried to reverse her decision to leave, only to discover a replacement had already been appointed. While her Head had expressed regret and kept her name on file for any future openings, it seemed her dream of a learning support role was gone. Then the first lockdown hit and she was overwhelmed with gratitude that she was able to be home to support her own children through the strain of home schooling. Spending extra time hunkered down at home with each of them had given opportunities for them all to express their emotions over the strain of the last year and the loss of their grandmother. She had watched and encouraged as they all evolved.

Molly had slowly come out of the quiet shell she had withdrawn into. The little terrapin Bobi had given her something of her own to lavish her soft heart's kindness on. She had basked in her mother's praise when her schoolwork was all completed quickly and neatly. Katie had realised how little her daughter had asked for and how little she had received in the past. Her quiet one had rediscovered her giggle.

Matt had been the most frustrated at being trapped at home until astonishingly Jack had rediscovered his own love of football and the two of them had spent hours kicking a ball through a makeshift goal in the garden and gleefully competing at keepie-uppies. Matt's school had been inconsistent in its approach to providing work and Katie had found herself supplementing and upgrading his studies. As a result, he was ahead rather than behind when schools reopened.

Jack had unravelled when first forced to work from home. Then with typical determination he had found a way to ensure he kept his earnings as high as previously. He was using Joan's old room as an office where he zoomed clients in peace and produced his presentations with no distractions. Freed from the constraints of a commute and client lunches he had found he had time on his hands. With no alternative but his family for company, he was forced into discovering how entertaining they were. He now enjoyed a far better relationship with each of his children. Along with the football, he had dug out all their old bikes and polished them up. He had ordered a special attachment for Lucy which was fixed to Katie's bike. While both of them pedalled, only Katie's hard work made a difference. It could have gone on

Jack's, but he was too busy racing Matt. The whole family would set off on sunny days and explore the lanes around their home. Jack had transformed indeed. When he came down those stairs, he shook off work and became the family man Katie had wished for without ever realising it. He could still be self-absorbed sometimes, although he had softened and mellowed in ways Katie could never have foreseen. She had worked harder at their marriage too and they were much closer. All it had taken was a tragedy, followed by a pandemic!

Lucy still suffered the occasional nightmare over the accident. Her arm ached in bad weather and she would frown and bite her lip whenever a car passed too fast. She had never asked to go to that park again. Katie's constant presence and reassuring cuddles were certainly making a difference, however she felt Lucy had not yet fully healed inside from the horror she had experienced. Something between them remained unspoken and Katie had no idea how to tackle it. Her mother would have quoted that time was a great healer and Katie clung to that belief. In practical ways she had been able to help Lucy. By closely observing her struggles with reading and writing Katie had realised it was likely her daughter was dyslexic. She used all her special needs teaching skills to help her improve and her knowledge of the assessment system to get Lucy some early interventions in place for when she returned to a school setting.

The driver who caused the accident had pleaded guilty and been sentenced to just five years for causing death by dangerous driving. They had at least been spared a trial, although Katie had seethed for a long time when told the judge had been lenient as it was a first and only offence. It was my only mother she had sobbed. Jack's attempt at comfort by reminding her that punishing the offender didn't change the outcome hadn't helped.

Lucy reached the graveside first. She glanced at her mother to check it was the right one. Katie nodded and they both looked down at the headstone. Joan had been buried next to her husband, but the wording reflected both their relationship and those she had left behind.

Joan Jessup
Wife of Colin
Cherished mother of Katie
Adored grandmother to Matthew,
Molly and Lucy

"Look Mummy there's my name!"
Katie smiled and read the wording out loud to her daughter.
"What's 'adored' mean?"
Katie bent down and looked straight into her daughter's eyes.
"It means you loved Grandma and she loved you more than anything in the whole world."
"It says Matt and Molly too."
"Yes, she loved them very much too."
Lucy nodded solemnly and bent down to pick up the vase Katie had left by the headstone. They walked up to the water butt where the Church warden kindly left a watering can to help fill vases.
"Can I pour the water Mummy?"
"Of course you can."
As she did water gushed out of the bottom and splashed all over Lucy's trousers. Lucy dropped it in surprise.
"I'm all wet Mummy!"
Katie bent down and felt the damage. One leg was soaked and with the wind chill she didn't want Lucy to stay outside too long.
"Let's get back to the car quickly and get you home and changed."
"But I haven't put my flowers in the pot."
Katie examined the vase. Despite being sold as a memorial vase it had clearly cracked in the cold weather.
"We won't be able to put any water in, but they will be OK for a day or two."
"I don't want them to die!" wailed Lucy.
"I'm sorry sweetheart there's not much I can do."
"Can we mend it?"
"I don't think so. Some things don't mend."
Katie looked at Lucy's sad face and watched as a tear trickled down her cheeks.

"It's only a few flowers, we can get another vase and come back with more."

"But these ones will be dead and I picked them specially for Grandma."

"I know, and she would love them, we can leave them here anyway."

"But…why won't it mend Mummy. Can't we fix it? Is it my fault? Did I do something wrong?"

Katie looked at Lucy's solemn face and realised there were other thoughts bubbling up behind her daughter's concern over the flowers.

"You didn't do anything wrong; it just broke."

"Was Grandma broken? Is that why she died?"

"Yes, that is one way of saying it. She was also very old."

"Only my arm was broken too but it mended. Why didn't Grandma's breaks mend?" Katie sighed and hugged her daughter tight.

"I don't know, I think her breaks were worse than yours."

"Because she stopped the car."

Those words hung on the air between them. Katie had never pressed Lucy for details of the accident. She had herself always believed her mother's actions were deliberate. Jack, while not agreeing, had allowed her to believe whatever gave her comfort. As there had been no trial the police had not pushed for information either. Now could be the moment Katie finally knew the truth. It had to be Lucy's choice to share.

"Do you want to talk about it? What happened that day? You don't have to. And nothing was ever your fault. You know that don't you?"

Lucy looked down at her shoes and then up at her mother. The words tumbled out.

"I was trying to show Grandma how to cross the road. On the zebra. She had forgotten. The car didn't stop. Grandma pushed me so it bumped her not me. I fell over on my arm. Grandma flew up in the air and landed all broken. I was scared."

Katie wrapped her tight in her arms.

"I know you were sweetheart, I'm so sorry it happened to you."

"Then lots of people came, policemen and ambulances and even you. Before you there was this nice lady who cuddled me and wouldn't let me look at Grandma." Katie knew there had been a woman who had helped her daughter. She had called the emergency services and had been cradling Lucy until Katie had arrived, running desperately towards them knowing she was too late…

"You know why Grandma did that don't you Lucy?" Lucy turned her tear-streaked face to her mother and shook her head slightly. "It's right there on her headstone. We just read it." She took Lucy by the hand and led her back to the grave.

"Look, the word you asked me to read, 'adored'. She loved you enough to stop a car even if it meant she died. She didn't mind as long as you were OK."

"Did you mind Mummy? Were you cross?"

Katie's mind flashed with images of the day. She had howled with despair and rage, unable to stop and comfort her child as her mother lay there all crumpled and bleeding.

"I was sad. I 'adored' my mother too and she was dead. I was angry that it had happened. Definitely not with you. I was angry with the man who drove the car and didn't stop." She paused and took a breath, "I was very glad Grandma saved you. Very grateful you were OK."

Lucy sniffed solemnly and reached up for a hug. They stood there for a moment, each lost in their own memories. Then carefully Lucy placed her flowers on the grave and they turned hand in hand and walked back to the car.

Acknowledgements

As I said in the foreword, this book grew from my own experience in dealing with my mother's dementia. She fought a brave battle but lost it in February 2022 and so this book is dedicated to her. However, I could not release it without acknowledging my amazing family, who made the nine years we cared for her more bearable. My husband Darrin, who could not be less like Jack if he tried and treated my mum with such tenderness. My grown-up children Michael and Heather, who rolled up their sleeves and pitched in to help, despite teenage pressures, exams and university deadlines. I will be forever grateful for the kindness and compassion they showed. And my littlest Jessica, who never knew Mum before her dementia began, but spent part of every day of her first 9 years playing with Grandma. From her I learned how to truly love without judgement. In our case dementia didn't win, love did.